Chronic Diseases in the year 2005

Chronic Diseases Scenario Committee
Chairman: Prof.Dr. A.F. Casparie

Chronic Diseases Research Team
Centre for Epidemiology
National Institute of Public Health and Environmental Protection
Senior researcher: Dr. H. Verkleij

Chronic Diseases in the year 2005

Volume 3
Scenarios on Rheumatoid Arthritis 1990-2005

Scenario report commissioned by the
Steering Committee on Future Health Scenarios

1994
Kluwer Academic Publishers
Dordrecht - Boston - London

Distributors

for the United States and Canada: Kluwer Academic Publishers,
P.O. Box 358, Accord Station, Hingham, MA 02018-0358, USA
for all other countries: Kluwer Academic Publishers Group, Distribution
Center, P.O. Box 322, 3300 AH Dordrecht, The Netherlands

Steering Committee
on Future Health Scenarios
P.O. Box 5406
2280 HK Rijswijk
The Netherlands
Telephone (31-70) 3407205

Translation of the Dutch original, `Chronische Ziekten in het jaar 2005, deel 3. Scenario's over reumatoide artritis 1990-2005' by Dr. J.W. Arriëns and J. Ross.

ISBN 0-7923-3367-5

PRINTED IN THE NETHERLANDS

TABLE OF CONTENTS

HOW TO USE THIS REPORT

This report is designed for a wide readership. Since it is not easy to summarize the results of the research in such a way as to produce a report that is interesting and readable for all, a brief guide on using the report is provided below.

Readers are advised to begin by reading the **Summary** (at the start of the report). This will familiarize them with the line of thought and the overall results of the research.

The report further consists of the following chapters:

- **Chapter 1** discusses the aims, limits and design of the research;
- **Chapter 2** provides a review of the current state of affairs in relation to rheumatoid arthritis in the Netherlands, followed by a comparison with other countries. The chapter also examines developments in the recent past and factors that could determine developments in this field in the future;
- **Chapter 3** provides an account of the main results of an enquiry into experts' expectations with respect to rheumatoid arthritis;
- **Chapter 4** presents three exploratory health scenarios and a policy scenario. The exploratory health scenarios are intended to provide an indication of the limits within which future developments (up to 2005) could take place, while the policy scenario examines the scope for influencing those developments;
- Finally **Chapter 5** draws conclusions from the research.

The diagnosis and treatment of rheumatoid arthritis are examined in an appendix.

The results of the research may be scanned by referring to the summary and sections 3.2 (results of the Delphi study) and 4.6 (conclusions relating to the scenarios). This might be followed by Chapter 5, which examines priority areas for government policy. The remaining chapters contain the most essential background information (Chapters 1 and 2).

SUMMARY

Aims and approach

In order to chart the way for long-term policies in the field of public health, the Dutch government needs to have the best possible insight into potential future trends and the problems to which these could give rise.

It was with a view to compiling a number of long-range studies that the independent Steering Committee on Future Health Scenarios (STG) was set up in 1983. In early 1988 the STG appointed a committee to study the likely future of chronic diseases. Three such diseases were selected: diabetes mellitus, CNSLD (chronic non-specific lung disease) and rheumatoid arthritis (a chronic disorder of the joints). These disorders were selected on the basis of their occurrence, duration and severity/intensity of care. The research is being conducted by the Department of Epidemiology of the National Institute of Public Health and Environmental Protection (RIVM) in close consultation with the committee.

This report contains the results of the study on rheumatoid arthritis (RA). In addition there is a large number of other rheumatic disorders that also affect a substantial proportion of the population. RA, however, is one of the most serious disorders, on which the most data are available. The other rheumatic disorders have consequently not been described in this report.

The report on diabetes mellitus appeared in March 1990 and that on CNSLD in December 1990. The series will be completed by a final report, in which the results of the three reports will be integrated (spring 1992) with a view to building up a general picture of chronic diseases.

The study centered on two questions based on a survey of the potential developments and the scope for intervention:

1. Survey of developments:
   - What are the likely trends in the number of RA-patients, the number and severity of the physical consequences, the quality of life and degree of care (including self-care)?

- What impact on these developments will demographic changes, changes in risk factors, developments in medical technology and changes in the structure of care and treatment have?
- What implications will this have for the uptake of care in the coming 10 to 15 years?

2. Scope for intervention:
   - What means does the government or other organizations and groups in society have to influence these developments, and what possible effects would these have?

The study was of an exploratory, not a predictive nature. It does not go beyond the year 2005. Given the numerous uncertainties and the pace of change, it was thought inadvisable to look ahead further than 15 years.

The study consisted of three parts. To begin with the current scale of the problem was examined and an analysis made, where possible, of trends in the recent past. A list of possible future developments was then drawn up. This was done with the aid of a Delphi study: a written questionnaire sent to a number of experts, conducted in two rounds, in which the participants remain anonymous to prevent them from influencing one another. The study concluded with a workshop. On the basis of this study a number of future scenarios were then drawn up differing from one another in terms of the assumed "autonomous" developments and the scope for influencing these developments by means of government action or by other groups in society. The number of patients up to the year 2005 was calculated with the aid of a computer model. Other implications of the various scenarios of the future in the year 2005 have largely been dealt with in descriptive terms.

Current scale of the problem

Rheumatoid arthritis is one of the most serious rheumatic disorders. The disease is characterized by the inflammation of a number of joints (polyarthritis). In many cases this is symmetrical, i.e. the same joints are affected in the left and right parts of the body. Although the disorder tends to be concentrated on the small joints of the hands and forefeet, the inflammation can occur in virtually any joint. Pain, stiffness and swelling of the joints are the main features, resulting in loss of function. In the end damage to the joints can lead to serious deformities (i.e. articular features) and functional impairments.

Apart from the effect on the joints, rheumatoid arthritis may be associated with a wide range of other features (i.e. extra-articular manifestations). While these phenomena are most common in the case of serious forms of rheumatoid arthritis, they may also provide the first symptom of the disease. Various organs, such as the heart, blood vessels, lungs and kidneys may be involved.

Rheumatoid arthritis generally manifests itself after puberty. The prevalence (i.e. the number of patients) rises with age. In overall terms the disorder is 2-3 times more frequent among women than men. A comparison of the occurrence of RA in the Netherlands with that abroad (in so far as this is possible) reveals that the Netherlands occupies an intermediate position. Figures supplies by the Nijmegen University Institute of General Practitioners suggest that some 93,500 RA-patients are at present known to general practitioners, or 0.6% of the Dutch population. The number of known patients with rheumatoid arthritis probably forms only a part of the total. Epidemiological studies indicate that, converted to 1990, the number of patients with rheumatoid arthritis should amount to around 139,000, or roughly 0.9% of the Dutch population. This would therefore mean that there are some 45,000 RA-patients who have never been diagnosed. It is however conceivable that some of these unknown patients will suffer from less serious complaints than the known patients.

The cause of rheumatoid arthritis remains the subject of considerable uncertainty. It is assumed that exposure to primary causative agents (e.g. bacteria or viruses) of individuals with a genetic predisposition can result in the onset of rheumatoid arthritis. This is associated with an abnormal reaction of the immune system, which plays a central role in the onset and progression of articular features and extra-articular manifestations that are characteristic of rheumatoid arthritis.

The treatment of RA-patients is essentially directed towards alleviating the discomfort caused by the symptoms as far as possible and arresting the progression of the disease. Depending on the symptoms, an appropriate medical therapy needs to be prescribed. In connection with side-effects and adjusting the medication, it is essential for the patient to be checked at regular intervals by a physician with sufficient expertise and experience in the field of rheumatic disorders. Apart from medication the treatment can consist of dosed rest, physiotherapy, occupational therapy and surgery. Good patient education is a vital precondition for the success of treatment.

The articular features and extra-articular manifestations of rheumatoid arthritis have a significant effect on the quality of life and medical consumption. Life expectancy is also affected by the disorder.

A survey has been conducted in the Netherlands into the median life expectancy (i.e. the point at which 50% of the individuals have died) of RA-patients in comparison with that of the general population. In the case of RA-patients receiving hospital/outpatient treatment, the life expectancy for males proved to be seven years shorter and that for females three years shorter.

The quality of life is influenced by articular features and extra-articular manifestations, as a result of which the patient is limited in managing daily activities. In addition the quality of life is affected by psychosocial problems. In a considerable number of patients rheumatoid arthritis results in marked uncertainty concerning the future, dependence on others, difficulty in maintaining social contacts, problems in relationships with partners, problems in family life and loss of hobbies. In a number of cases this can lead to depression. The negative impact of rheumatoid arthritis on the physical and psychosocial functioning is one of the causes of the higher degree of sickness absence and employment disability of rheumatoid arthritis patients compared with the Dutch population as a whole.

Rheumatoid arthritis results in an appreciable uptake of health care (i.e. medical consumption). Figures for the period 1988-1989 indicate that at least 159,000 GP consultations, at least 140,000 specialist consultations (of which 80,000-98,000 with a rheumatologist), 4,900 hospital admissions, over 121,000 hospital patient days and at least 360,000 nursing days in nursing homes were attributable (in full or in part) to rheumatoid arthritis.

The figures presented form an *absolute baseline* for the true medical consumption as these are often based on data in which RA was the primary diagnosis. This takes no account of the fact that RA is often the cause of or a contributory factor towards medical consumption without being specifically mentioned in the medical records. The difference can sometimes involve a factor of two to three. On account of lack of data not all centres specifically concerned with rheumatic disorders have been included in the figures. At the risk of stating the obvious, it may be noted that these figures relate only to RA. Had the figures covered all rheumatic diagnoses the numbers would have been much higher.

Developments in recent years

A number of significant developments have taken place in both medical and surgical treatments in recent decades.

The arsenal of drugs has been expanded but also of relevance are the improvements that have helped reduce the side-effects. Further improvements may be expected in the existing drugs in the coming years (namely fewer side-effects), while new drugs will also become available. The consequences of the disease can also be limited by suppressing its activity at an early stage.

Surgery makes an important contribution. Some years ago it was only possible to immobilize a destroyed joint (arthrodesis). In the late 1960s it became possible to replace the joint with an artificial one (arthroplasty). To begin with this was limited to the hip, followed later by the knee. Recently shoulder-joints have also been replaced and protheses are being developed for the ankle and elbow. On account of the limited life of the artificial joints, joint-replacement operations were initially confined to older patients. Improvements in the quality of the protheses and operating techniques mean that younger patients can now also be operated on. Surgery of the hand occupies a special place. On account of the complex anatomy, this form of surgery is generally carried out by plastic surgeons.

Possible future developments

In order to reduce the wide range of future possibilities and the scope for intervention to manageable proportions, four types of scenarios have been developed on the basis of the results of the Delphi study (Table 1).

Table 1 Formulated scenarios

Surveys of developments:	- Demographic scenario
	Reference scenario
	- Alternative scenarios
Potential for intervention	- Policy scenario

The first three (exploratory) scenarios are designed to provide an indication of the range within which future developments are likely to take place. In partly statistical and partly descriptive terms, these scenarios describe likely trends, subject to varying assumptions, in the number of RA-patients, the number and severity of articular features and extra-articular manifestations, the quality of life and medical consumption. The policy scenario examines the possibility for influencing these developments.

Demographic scenario
As old people are more susceptible to chronic disorders such as RA, demographic trends (especially ageing) play a highly important role in forecasting the likely course of such disorders. The probable number of patients in 2005 has been calculated with the aid of a mathematical model known as the "static" model.

The calculations for the static model indicate that the likely demographic changes will result in a 21% increase in the number of known RA-patients between 1990 and 2005 (see Table 2).

It is not clear to what extent this increase is a real one, as the static model does not make allowance for on-going trends from the past. The development of a dynamic model, in which allowance is made for trends from the past, did not prove possible for rheumatoid arthritis on account of the lack of reliable data on the inflow of new patients (i.e. incidence) and outflow of known patients (mortality/recovery).

If demographic changes only are included in the model, the medical consumption **as a result of** rheumatoid arthritis rises in line with the number of patients. On account of the process of ageing, the medical consumption as a result of rheumatoid arthritis for those forms of care for which there is a particular demand among patients in the older age categories (i.e. outpatient care and nursing home care) will rise disproportionately. Although no reliable data were available, it may be assumed that the same applies to district nursing care and home help.

Reference scenario
The reference scenario occupies a special place, being largely based on the insights of the experts interviewed in the Delphi study with respect to the

most probable developments up to the year 2005. The panel was asked to make a judgement independent of demographic changes, so that the responses could be interpreted in "pure" form. Tables 3 and 4 provide a summary of the expectations in simplified form.

A significant expectation is the fact that according to the Delphi respondents, the incidence (i.e. the number of new patients per 1,000 inhabitants in a particular age group) will remain unchanged. The respondents also expect an increase in the percentage of patients actually diagnosed as such (see Table 3). At present it is assumed that only 50% of all RA-patients are diagnosed, while by 2005 it is expected that 60% of all RA-patients will be known to their general practitioners. An estimate of the increase in the number of patients with RA is provided in Table 2 in the light of this assumption.

Table 2 Estimated number of patients with rheumatoid arthritis (x 1,000) in 1990 and 2005 known to their general practitioner given an unchanged (demographic scenario) and a changed rate of diagnosis (reference scenario)

Scenario	1990	2005	1990-2005 Increase absolute	%
Demographic scenario*	93.5	113	19.5	21
Reference scenario**	93.5	135.5	42	45

* Unchanged rate of diagnosis of 50%.

** Modified rate of diagnosis of 50% in 1990 rising to 60% in 2005; the impact of the anticipated (extra) increase in life expectancy on the number of RA-patients has not been calculated but is in all probability low.

The result of the increase in the rate of diagnosis (combined with the consequences of the demographic trends) is a 45% increase in the number of known RA-patients in 2005 in relation to 1990. Caution is certainly in order when it comes to interpreting the extent of the increase in the diagnostic rate, since there is a large spread in the respondents' views on the present rate of diagnosis and the likely rate in 2005.

The Delphi respondents expect no change or even a fall in the occurrence and severity of articular features. No changes in the incidence and severity of the extra-articular manifestations are expected. Complications could however arise more frequently as a result of the treatment in the coming 15 years. The quality of life will improve somewhat and the life expectancy will increase by roughly one (additional) year in comparison with the general population (see Table 3).

Table 3 Summary of the main results of the Delphi study: developments to the year 2005 given unchanged demographic trends (N = 17 to 30)

Variable	Change
Incidence (age-specific)	0
Rate of diagnosis	+
Occurrence and severity of articular features	0/-
Occurrence and severity of extra-articular manifestations	0
Occurrence of complications resulting from treatment	+
Quality of life	+/0
Life expectancy	+/0

Explanation of codes: + = increase; 0 = no change; - = decrease

According to the Delphi respondents the percentage of patients in primary health care and receiving out-patient treatment will rise due to shifts in health care. The percentage of patients receiving hospital and nursing home care will decline slightly while the proportion being looked after in rest homes will remain roughly unchanged (see Table 4).

The quantity of care demanded per day by an "average" RA-patient receiving treatment in primary health care or from hospital, outpatient, nursing home or rest home care will increase (see Table 4).

Table 4 Summary of the main results of the Delphi Study concerning the expected demand for care: developments to the year 2005 given unchanged demographic trends, incidence, life expectancy and diagnostic rates (N = 31)

	Percentage of RA patients receiving care	Demand for care per patient receiving care per day
Primary		
general practitioner	+/0	+/0
district nursing	+/0	+/0
physiotherapy	+/0	+/0
ergotherapy	+	+
family care	+	+
Secondary		
outpatient	+	+
hospital	0/-	+/0
Tertiary		
specialist rheumatology hospital	+/0/-	+/0/-
nursing home	0/-	+/0
rest home	0	+/0

Explanation of codes: + = increase; 0 = no change; - = decrease

Alternative scenarios

In order to chart the effects of other possible developments, contrasting or alternative scenarios have been developed. These differ from the reference scenario in terms of the underlying assumptions. In particular, these concern developments about which there is marked uncertainty as to whether they will in fact occur or what direction the effects will take. Two types of alternative scenarios have been developed, a scenario on case-finding and one on spending cuts.

By case-finding is meant the active identification in general practice of as yet undiagnosed rheumatoid arthritis patients. The case-finding scenario makes a numerical estimate of the number of diagnosed RA-patients in 2005 in the extreme case that (nearly) all patients with RA will be diagnosed at an early stage in the next 15 years.

The spending-cuts scenario provides a description of the consequences that could occur in the years ahead if major cuts in health care were enforced on account of the weakness of the economy.

How to proceed?

The scope for favourably influencing developments such as those outlined in the exploratory scenarios is examined below. It will be evident that limiting the anticipated increase in the number of RA-patients, reducing the number and severity of articular features and extra-articular manifestations and improving the quality of life will require a great deal of effort and investment in the fields of care, research and education.

Policy scenario

The possibilities for tackling the RA problem in the coming years are described in the policy scenario. The central aspects dealt with in the policy scenario are listed in Table 5. The scenario committee is of the view that attention needs to be devoted to all these aspects.

Table 5 Content of the policy scenario

a. Prevention:	- Fundamental research
b. Medical care:	- Expansion in care - Health care innovations
c. Social functioning	

a. Policies aimed at prevention

The cause of RA is still insufficiently understood for successful preventive measures to be taken. Progress is at the same time being made towards a greater understanding of the disease and research into the cause of RA deserves to be vigorously expanded. Particular efforts should be made to encourage research in those areas where experts consider that marked progress can be made. In particular, major advances could be made in understanding the mechanism of the immune response and the latter's connection with genetic predisposition and primary causative agents (e.g. viruses and bacteria). The possibility that the improved understanding of the immune response mechanism could be used in the primary prevention of RA before the year 2005, thus appreciably reducing the incidence before that year, may however be ruled out as the effects will not become evident until much later in the future.

Possibilities for improved secondary prevention - defined as the prevention of irreversible damage, e.g. to the joints - will, however, in all probability emerge at an earlier stage. Improvements in understanding of the immune mechanism will enable the immune system among RA-patients to be influenced more effectively by means of medical treatment. The progression of RA can consequently be positively influenced, thus saving a good deal of suffering. Insight into the effectiveness of such intervention will, in particular, need to be provided by longer-term patient-related scientific research.

b. Medical care

Expansion of medical care

For a number of reasons marked priority needs to be placed on the expansion of medical care:

1. In the first place the number of patients with RA will increase in the coming years on account of the ageing of the population and the increase in the diagnostic rate. On the basis of the ageing process a 21% increase in the number of diagnosed patients is anticipated in the period 1990-2005 (demographic scenario). If the future demand for care is to be satisfied the provision of care will need to expand commensurately. The process of ageing will mean that the number of older patients rises disproportionately, so that extra expansion will be required for those forms of care specially directed towards this category (i.e. outpatient care, nursing home care and - despite the lack of reliable data - district nursing and family care).
2. If account is also taken of the anticipated increase in the diagnostic rate, this could lead to an increase in the number of RA-patients of around 45% (reference scenario). The additional increase will in all probability consist of patients generally suffering from less serious forms of RA. This increase may be expected to place particular demand

on outpatient rheumatology clinics, general practitioners, physiotherapists and drug consumption.

3. In addition, independently of the increase in the number of patients, the percentage of patients receiving treatment at primary level and in outpatient rheumatology clinics will rise still further, as will the demand for care per patient in these forms of care (reference scenario).
4. Finally an expansion in care will be required in order to eliminate the present shortfall of RA care in relation to the demand. This applies especially to specialist rheumatological care. An application has been made to the Hospital Facilities Council for an advisory report on the scope of care provisions in the field of rheumatology. The extent of the shortfall is currently being investigated by the Catholic University of Brabant in collaboration with the University of Groningen, covering not just RA but also other rheumatic disorders. A report recently published by the Hospital Facilities Council also identifies the shortfall in the orthopaedic field.

Health care innovations

In the light of the present problems being encountered in the provision of RA care, attention also needs to be devoted to improving the quality of care. Measures to improve the quality of care are likely to lead fairly quickly to visible results. In particular, greater attention needs to be devoted to promoting the level of expertise among carers, especially general practitioners (e.g. by improvements in basic training and the development and possibly compulsory introduction of further training courses, etc.). At the same time, however, the standard of knowledge among other carers (such as district nurses, home-helps and rheumatologists) needs to be improved in certain areas. The training needs to pay specific attention to socio-medical and psychological aspects. An important priority in promoting the level of expertise is to provide carers with sufficient experience in dealing with the problems faced by RA-patients.

Attention needs to be devoted to improving the cooperation between primary and secondary health care with respect to RA. One solution would consist of the appointment of rheumatology teams based around a rheumatologist and a hospital/community rheumatology nurse. Apart from the treatment and counselling of RA-patients they act as case-coordinator and exercise a consultative function with respect to other care providers (i.e. the transfer of expertise).

c. Social functioning
In view of the fact that RA-patients remain in a situation of social disadvantage, it is important to encourage measures to improve their ability to function in society. Employment opportunities for RA-patients could be improved by the more effective enforcement of the Handicapped Employees (Employment) Act (WAGW), with sanctions against uncooperative employers. The provision of more and improved information to employers, personnel officers, medical examiners and Joint Medical Service (GMD) and Industrial Insurance Administration Office (GAK) doctors could make a contribution in this respect. Other measures to improve the social functioning of RA-patients include the relaxation and simplification of the regulations concerning ergotherapy and the application procedures for appliances and adaptations, the availability of occupational therapists and "adaptable" housing, etc. Measures to influence public opinion about the relationship between rheumatic disorders (including RA) and handicapped persons (e.g. by public education and information) could play an important role in this respect.

Provision of information and scientific research

By way of policy support, improved information provision and the expansion of scientific research are required. The Chronic Diseases scenario study indicated that the quantity and quality of the available data on RA were rather limited. A number of recommendations are therefore provided below on the way in which the provision of information could be improved and the form that the scientific research might take.

Improvement of the provision of information
To a greater extent than (for example) in the scenario study "Accidents and Traumatology", the Chronic Diseases Scenario Committee encountered a lack of reliable data in the field of RA. This meant that even drawing up a general picture of the field was a difficult exercise. The same applied to diabetes mellitus and CNSLD but even more markedly in the case of RA.

Where data were lacking, a choice had to be made in the background chapter (Chapter 2) between the presentation of general impressions and leaving estimates out altogether. It was decided in favour of the latter, i.e. circumscribed reporting based on empirical data, since this was an initial, detailed presentation of the field and it was therefore important for this to be as firmly based as possible.

An important set of records is the Standard Diagnosis Register of Rheumatic Diseases (SDR) initiated by the TNO Committee for Rheumatology Research in 1977, which contains information on outpatient rheumatological care.

There remain however significant deficiencies in the registration of RA. The most notable of these are:

- A lack of recent reliable (trend) data on the incidence and prevalence of RA in the population. The most recent survey was the EPOZ study conducted in 1975-1978.
- There is a lack of reliable data on the incidence of RA in general practice. The populations examined are too small to permit well-founded statements to be made.
- In so far as they are available, the data on the incidence of articular features and extra-articular manifestations of RA are inadequate, particularly as regards their development in individual patients (i.e. the natural course).
- There is a lack of reliable (trend) data on the medical consumption as a result of this disorder. In so far as such data are recorded it tends, for various reasons, to suffer from underreporting (e.g. in the case of the LMR/SIG).
- There is a lack of reliable (trend) data on the mortality as a result of RA. There are good reasons to assume a substantial measure of underreporting in the CBS cause-of-death statistics.

For the purposes of policy formulation, the setting up of continuous monitoring projects to chart the scale of the RA problem is therefore a top priority.

In contrast to the situation with respect to diabetes mellitus and CNSLD, the even greater lack of reliable information means that it was decided not to be feasible to examine the costs associated at the present time and in 15 years time with the care of RA. Further research is required in this area.

The importance of scientific research
One important function of the Chronic Diseases scenario study is to identify gaps in the research field. The fact that an absence of reliable

information was identified in relation to so many aspects means that a large number of potential research topics can be generated. This in turn makes it essential to design a coherent package of such topics, thereby providing RA research policy with a clearer framework. The TNO Committee for Rheumatology Research has also identified a number of obstacles towards scientific research in its report "Naar een nieuw tijdsgewricht" (Towards a New Juncture) (CR-TNO 1990). These obstacles have been incorporated in the topics outlined below. We shall confine ourselves to the most important topics:

Monitoring:

- Conducting an epidemiological **population study**. This enables insight to be obtained into the current scale of RA (and comparisons to be made with previous epidemiological studies). Moreover, this would enable the patients known to general practitioners to be compared with those newly discovered as a result of the population study. In order to analyse the determinants for the prognosis for RA, such a study would need to be longitudinal. It would also need to be set up along the same lines as other international studies in this field.
- The setting up and continuation of continuous monitoring projects in **a large number of general practices** needs to be coupled with scientific research in order to obtain a reliable insight into trends in RA and the (trends in the) development of articular features, extra-articular manifestations and medical consumption. The aim in doing so would be to enable an overall assessment to be made as to whether the RA problem was growing or declining. Once again this would need to be conducted along the same lines as international studies in this field.
- Efforts should be made to increase the number of rheumatologists participating in the SDR so that **outpatient care** can be properly charted at national level. There would also be a strong case for integration with the SIG's outpatient surveillance system (POLIS).

Prevention:

- Research into the causes of RA needs to be considerably expanded (section 4.5, the prevention scenario), with a view not just to primary prevention but also to secondary prevention.

Treatment and care:

- Research into the accessibility of rheumatological care, including professional help by rehabilitation specialists, physiotherapists, occupational therapists, rheumatology nurses, general practitioners, district nurses and home helps (this is currently being investigated for rheumatology and has just been investigated for orthopaedics).

- Research into the help actually provided by the patient's immediate support circle and other volunteers, as well as research into the consequences of the provision of such help on those close to the patient (e.g. over-burdening).
- Research into the accessibility of adaptations and aids (e.g. in the work situation).
- Research into the effects, accessibility and quality of the information provided by patients' associations, Health Information and Education (GVO) consultants and professional carers.
- Research into the quality of life of RA-patients. This needs to include an investigation into optimal methods of coping with the disease. Aspects of the quality of life need to be taken into consideration in the evaluation of particular developments and measures.
- Research in the field of medication. This may be regarded as a natural extension of the research into the causes of RA. Greater insight into the immune mechanism will enable more selective treatment. In addition research is required into the long-term effects of medication.
- Research into the role of physiotherapy. Are there certain categories of RA-patients for whom a particular therapy is effective and what then is the effect?
- Research into the present and future role of specialist rheumatological care.

There are various fields in which initiatives and research plans could be stimulated. The Committee for Rheumatological Research notes that the training of researchers concentrating on basic and patient-related research is one of the major problems at the present time, as is the career planning of such researchers, in view of the short-term nature of most research projects.

Comparison of scenarios in the report "Towards a new Juncture"

In its report "Towards a new Juncture" the TNO Committee for Rheumatology Research has drawn up a number of scenarios for rheumatic disorders (including RA). The report formulates objectives with respect to rheumatology services, rheumatological education and rheumatological research (including their financing). Three successive scenarios have been drawn up. These scenarios have in common that the infrastructure should be improved by reducing the dependence on collection-box funds and by arranging permanent financing. Scenario I, "Down to the bone", is a modest, conservative and consolidating scenario. Scenario II, "Movement", provides for a gradual growth in all aspects of rheumatology (university and otherwise). With respects to rheumatological care this means that the present shortfall in care facilities needs to be eliminated and that allowance needs to be made for a growing requirement for care. Education and research need to be encouraged in this context. Scenario III, "Towards a new Juncture", seeks in addition to put forward direct practical solutions for the problem of the accessibility of care.

It is notable that although the Committee for Rheumatological Research approaches the issue from a different angle (namely improvements in the infrastructure for research, whereas the scenario committee's point of departure consisted of likely developments in the number of patients and the burden of care), the aspects of care, education and research as specified in scenario III of the Committee for Rheumatological Research are reflected in the various themes of the policy scenario for rheumatoid arthritis as drawn up by the Scenario Committee for Chronic Diseases (Table 5).

There are also differences. The Committee for Rheumatological Research's scenarios relates to rheumatology in general, including rheumatoid arthritis, and to the period 1990-1995. The scenarios are oriented towards the introduction of concrete plans. The desirable expansions have been formulated in quantitative terms, with an indication of the financial consequences and the necessary organizational frameworks. The Committee's scenarios do not, however, specifically take up the social functioning of RA-patients. By contrast, the Scenario Committee did decide to devote separate attention to this aspect in its policy scenario for rheumatoid arthritis patients. The Scenario Committee's scenarios also cover a longer period, namely 1990-2005. By indicating the growth in the number of patients and the uptake of care in the various scenarios, a number of possible policy choices and the associated costs are implicitly brought into focus. The demographic scenario involves the least marked increase in costs. The reference scenario will presumably involve greater costs (as the net outcome of cuts and extra spending), while implementation of the policy scenario would involve the greatest cost.

Formulation of a coherent policy

The main impulses for new developments in the field of rheumatology have come from the health care system and the field of scientific research, although the government has also paid a part.

Within the field of heath care various associations are active in the field of rheumatic diseases, including RA. The National Rheumatology Fund and the Netherlands Association for the Control of Rheumatological Diseases (NVRB) may be regarded as a functional entity whose aim is to promote control of rheumatic disorders in the Netherlands. The Committee for Rheumatology Research of the TNO Health Research Division coordinates the rheumatology research. This committee originally set up by the Ministry of Health (WVC) also serves as an advisory body for the NVRB with respect to the scientific research subsidized by the latter organization.

In addition there is the Netherlands Federation of Associations of Patients with Rheumatic Disorders comprising 16,500 members from 92 local patients' associations, which publishes the monthly magazine "On the Move"; the Netherlands Association of Rheumatologists; the Netherlands Association for Rheumatological Surgery (NVRC), known as the Netherlands Rheumatoid Arthritis Surgical Society (NERASS) until 18 March 1991; the Netherlands Association of Nurses and Carers in Rheumatology; and the National Working Group for Physiotherapy in Rheumatic Diseases.

The tripartite consultations between the Netherlands Association for Rheumatalogical Control, the Netherlands Federation of Associations with Patients with Rheumatic Disorders and the Netherlands Association of Rheumatologists (set up in 1983) bring together the various parties for the purpose of exchanging information, consultation and joint policy. Intensive cooperation between all the aforementioned organizations involved in the care of rheumatic disorders is vital for the formulation of a coherent RA policy. Clear steps in this direction are being taken by workers in the health care field as part of the follow up to the report "Towards a New Juncture."

Rheumatic disorders have been the object of government interest on a number occasions in recent years. High priority has, for example been assigned to rheumatology research on the basis of the recommendations of the Science Policy Advisory Council (1983) and the Health Council

(1985) in the Health Research Promotion Programme (SGO) published in 1985. This was subsequently elaborated as the initial element of the Promotion Programme, in which respect a programme was drawn up for the years 1986-1990. The Rheumatic Disorders Policy Document published as one of the annexes to the draft Discussion Document on Health Policy published in 1989 by the Ministry of Welfare, Health and Cultural Affairs also devoted separate attention to rheumatic disorders, formulating a number of policy intentions. The "Chronic Diseases" scenario study is a further policy initiative by the government in the field of rheumatic disorders, especially RA.

In its policy document "Working Towards Innovations in Health Care" the present government has announced a number of significant policy intentions, including the allocation of priority to chronic diseases. The Chronic Diseases Policy Memorandum was submitted to the Lower House in early 1991. This memorandum identifies a number of obstacles applying to a number of chronic disorders, including RA. The memorandum was formulated on the basis of talks conducted with a number of organizations. These problems and obstacles - which especially reflect the views of patients' organizations - formed the input for the National Committee for the Chronically Ill set up in mid 1991, which has not just an advisory role but also a number of executive responsibilities. The main thrust of the draft Discussion Document on Health Policy was further elaborated in the Health Policy Document submitted to Parliament in mid-1991.

Of particular importance is the fact that the government is in the process of developing an integral policy plan with respect to chronic diseases in consultation with health-care workers. In this respect rheumatoid arthritis and rheumatic disorders in general should occupy an important place in view of the scale and severity of the problem. The research and education policy needs to be examined in detail in the policy plan as many questions remain unanswered. In order to improve the standard of the research and education, an established infrastructure is first required.

Conclusion

The research makes it clear that policy-makers cannot depend on favourable "autonomous" developments. The provision of an adequate amount and standard of care for a growing number of RA-patients will require substantial efforts on the part of governmental authorities, care providers, patients and society in general. The same applies even more to reducing the scale of the problem by prevention and eliminating the shortfall of care in the field of rheumatic diseases.

A special recommendation of the Steering Committee on Future Health Scenarios is that there should be a continuation of the RA scenario study in the form of an updating study, so that a document would become available in a number of years concerning the developments that had taken place with respect to RA. On the basis of the new data it would then be possible to determine whether the actual developments were diverging from those in the reference scenario. The scenario most closely in line with the actual course of events would then provide an impression of the possible consequences, thus providing a basis for the adjustment of policy goals.

Photograph captions

Many patients with rheumatoid arthritis develop more or less serious deformities of the hands, with pain and loss of function (photo top right). Some of these can end up as severe deformities (photo bottom right).

Improved treatment possibilities at an early stage reduce the number of patients with moderate/severe deformities, but highly serious deformities still occur at the present time, not just in the hands but also in other joints. In many cases partial treatment of highly serious deformities is now possible.

Photographs: Paul Weise, Medische Spectrum Twente, 1991

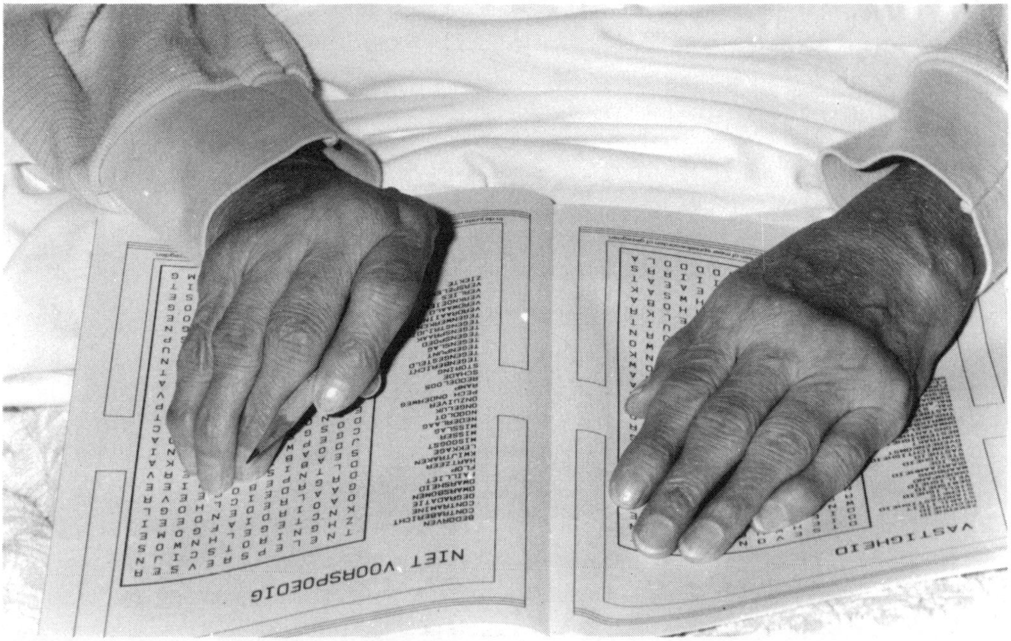
NIET VOORSPOEDIG
VASTIGHEID

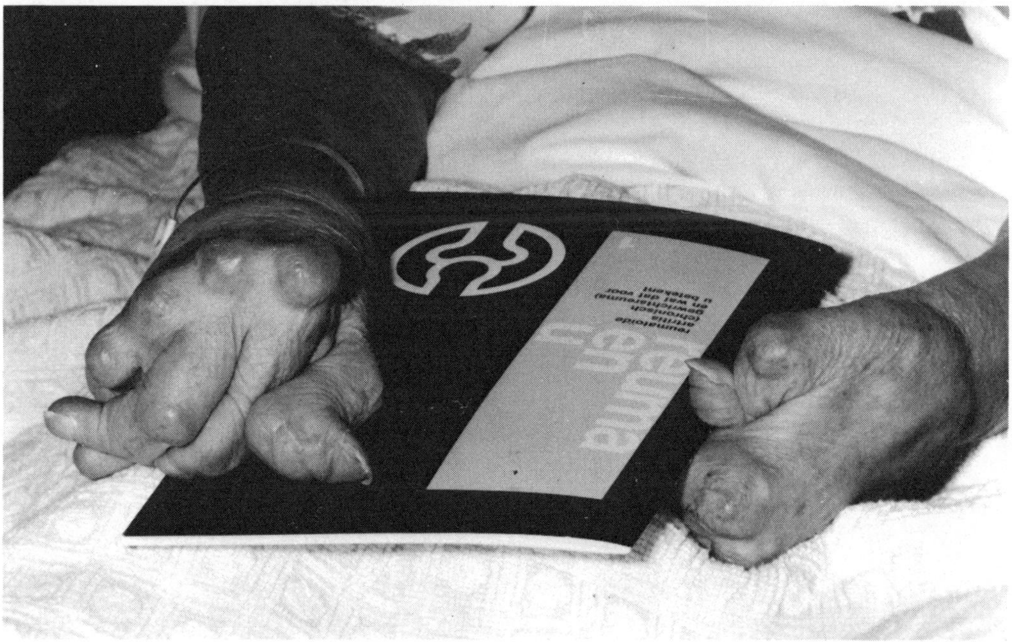

1 INTRODUCTION

1.1 For whom is this report intended?

This report contains the result of the study into rheumatoid arthritis (RA). In addition there are numerous other rheumatic disorders which also affect a large element of the population. RA, however, is one of the most serious disorders, and one on which more data are available than on most. The other rheumatic disorders have therefore not been described in this report.

The study is a long-term survey to the year 2005. As will be evident from the content of the report, major efforts will be required in order to minimize the increase in the problem of rheumatoid arthritis as a result of the ageing of the population. Measures will be required in order to "absorb" the growing number of patients with rheumatoid arthritis adequately in the health care system and to limit the consequences of rheumatoid arthritis in daily life. The report sets out to stimulate thinking about the appropriate strategies required.

In doing so the report is directed to all the parties concerned in these policy efforts. The problem affects not just the government and politicians but also the health care system, individual professional practitioners, patients' associations and scientific researchers concerned with the prevention and consequences of this disease and the provision of help for rheumatoid arthritis patients. The problem also touches society in general in terms of the appropriate responses to patients with rheumatoid arthritis and their handicaps. This report is designed for everyone who feels involved in the campaign to help curb this major health problem.

1.2 Aims of this study

The official title of the long-range research that forms the subject of this report is "The future burden of chronic diseases for Dutch society: scenarios for diabetes mellitus, CNSLD and rheumatoid arthritis 1990-2005". The study was commissioned by the Steering Committee on Future Health Scenarios, which was set up in 1983 by the State Secretary of the Ministry of Welfare, Health and Cultural Affairs. The Committee's terms of reference were to explore possible future developments in the field of health and health care. To this end the Steering Committee set up expert committees in various fields, assisted by research teams, in order to carry out a number of scenario projects. Studies of this kind have now been carried out in the fields of cardiovascular disease, cancer, ageing, medical technology, accidents and traumatology, mental health and employment and health. Scenario projects are currently under way concerning basic health care and the organization of primary health care while a feasibility study is being conducted into a scenario project concerning physical handicaps.

The results of these surveys of future developments play a role in the long-term policies of the Dutch government. The results of the completed scenario projects have, for example, been incorporated in the draft Discussion Document on Health Policy (1) issued by the Ministry of Welfare, Health and Cultural Affairs in mid-1989 as a follow up to its Report 2000 (2). The analysis in the scenario reports of the present health situation and the relevant determinants has provided the basis for the formulation of a number of (reasonably) concrete proposals for prevention and supporting policies. In the case of cardiovascular diseases, cancer and accidents and traumatology, a number of quantitative health targets were also formulated.

The new government which took office in November 1989 decided to shift the emphasis in health care policy. The Health Care Innovation Policy Document (3) outlines the most important policy lines and measures which the government intends introducing in the coming years. In early 1991 the Chronic Diseases Policy Memorandum was submitted to the Lower House (4), under which high priority was assigned to the care of chronic disorders. For this reason the National Committee for the Chronically Ill was set up on 29 May 1991. This committee, consisting of external experts, will advise on government policy and will also undertake a number of executive tasks. The results of the present scenario report will in all probability be used in the work of the National Committee and future policy documents on chronic diseases to formulate more specific health targets for these disorders.

In close consultation with the scenario committee of the same name, the "Chronic Diseases" scenario study has been carried out by the Department of Epidemiology of the National Institute of Public Health and Environmental Protection (RIVM) in Bilthoven. The research design and structure of the report closely follow that of previous scenario studies, especially "Accidents and Traumatology" (5).

Chronic diseases have been selected as the subject for a scenario study as these are characteristic diseases of our time, in the same way that infectious diseases were characteristic of the last century. Chronic diseases may be defined in various ways; generally these cover diseases from which people suffer long term or with which they are recurrently affected over a period of years (6). On account of their severity, they involve long-term limitations and impose a lasting burden on the health care system in terms of treatment and/or prevention (2, 7). It is on these two latter aspects that the scenario study focuses.

The "Chronic Diseases" scenario study (concentrating in this report on RA) poses two central questions concerning likely trends and the way in which these may be influenced:

1. Analysis of likely trends:
   - What are the likely trends in the number of RA-patients, the number and severity of the physical consequences, the quality of life and degree of care/self-care?
   - What impact on these trends will demographic changes, changes in risk factors, developments in medical technology and changes in the structure of care and treatment have?
   - What indications will this have in terms of demands made on health care over the next 10 to 15 years?
2. Scope for intervention:
   - What means does the government or other organizations and groups in society have to influence these developments and what possible effect would these have?

Given the speed of change in this field and the large margin of uncertainty that has to be taken into account, it became clear at an early stage that it would not be possible to make considered judgments for a period greater than 10 to 15 years. For this reason the survey has not been taken beyond the year 2005.

1.3 Delimitation of the field: diabetes mellitus, CNSLD and rheumatoid arthritis

Chronic diseases are many and varied, which makes it impossible to lump them together. One of the first questions that therefore needs to be answered in conducting a study of chronic diseases is to define which diseases are to be regarded as chronic and which are to be included in the survey. Since scenario studies had already been conducted for cardiovascular diseases and cancer, which account for the bulk of total mortality, it was clear that attention should now be directed towards a number of chronic diseases that are less important in terms of mortality but which are a major factor in morbidity.

At the request of the STG, the Netherlands Institute of Preventive Health Care (NIPG/TNO) carried out a preliminary study with a view to making a considered choice. On the basis of three criteria - occurrence, average duration and severity/intensity of care - the researchers in this institute recommended that scenario studies be set up in the fields of diabetes mellitus and CNSLD (chronic non-specific lung disease). As a third disorder the choice was narrowed down to rheumatoid arthritis and multiple sclerosis (6.7), with the STG's choice ultimately falling on rheumatoid arthritis as it is a more frequently encountered disorder.

This report discusses only rheumatoid arthritis. While it is emphasized that there are also numerous other rheumatic disorders, RA is one of the most serious disorders, on which the most data are available. Separate reports have appeared on diabetes mellitus (9) and CNSLD (10). The series will conclude with a final report integrating the results of the three reports (spring 1992).

1.4 Rheumatoid arthritis

Rheumatoid arthritis is one of the most serious rheumatic disorders. It is characterized by the inflammation of a number of joints (polyarthritis). In many cases this is symmetrical, i.e. the same joints are affected in the left and right parts of the body. Although the disorder tends to be concentrated on the small joints of the hands and forefeet, the inflammation can occur in virtually any joint. Pain, stiffness and swelling of the joints are the main features, resulting in loss of function. In the end damage to the joints can lead to serious deformities (i.e. **articular features/symptoms**) with a marked loss of functional capacity (see section 2.2.2).

Apart from the effect on the joints, rheumatoid arthritis may be associated with a wide range of other **extra-articular manifestations**. While these phenomena are most common in the case of serious forms of rheumatoid arthritis, they may also provide the first symptom of the disorder. Various organs, such as the heart, blood vessels, lungs and kidneys may be involved (see section 2.2.2).

Rheumatoid arthritis generally manifests itself after puberty. The prevalence (i.e. the number of patients) rises with age. In overall terms the disorder is 2-3 times more frequent among women than men. Figures supplies by the Nijmegen University Institute of General Practitioners suggest that some 93,500 RA-patients are at present known to general practitioners, or 0.6% of the Dutch population. The **number of known patients** with rheumatoid arthritis probably forms only a part of the total. Epidemiological studies indicate that, converted to 1990, the number of patients with rheumatoid arthritis should amount to around 139,000, or roughly 0.9% of the Dutch population. This would therefore mean that there are some 45,000 RA-patients who have never been diagnosed as such. It is however conceivable that some of these unknown patients will suffer from less serious complaints than the known patients (see section 2.2.1.2).

The cause of rheumatoid arthritis remains the subject of considerable uncertainty. It is assumed that exposure to **primary causative agents** (e.g. bacteria or viruses) of individuals with an immunogenetic **predisposition** can result in the onset of rheumatoid arthritis. This is associated with an abnormal reaction of the immune system, which plays a central role in the onset and progression of articular and extra-articular disorders that are characteristic of rheumatoid arthritis (see section 2.2.1.4).

The **treatment** of RA-patients is essentially directed towards alleviating the discomfort caused by the symptoms as far as possible and arresting the progression of the disease. Depending on the complaints, an adequate medical therapy needs to be prescribed. In connection with side-effects and adjusting the medication, it is essential for the patient to be checked at regular intervals by a physician with sufficient expertise and experience in this field. Apart from medication the treatment can consist of dosed rest, physiotherapy, occupational therapy and surgery. Good patient education is a vital precondition for the success of treatment (see Appendix 1).

The articular features and extra-articular manifestations of rheumatoid arthritis have a significant effect on the quality of life and medical consumption. Life expectancy is also affected by the disorder.

A survey has been conducted in the Netherlands into the median **life expectancy** (i.e. the point at which 50% of the individuals have died) of RA-patients in comparison with that of the general population. In the case of RA-patients receiving hospital/outpatient treatment, the life expectancy for males proved to be seven years shorter and that for females three years shorter (2.2.1.3).

The **quality of life** is influenced by articular features and extra-articular manifestations, as a result of which the patient is limited in managing daily activities. In addition the quality of life is affected by psychosocial problems. In a considerable number of patients rheumatoid arthritis results in marked uncertainty concerning the future, dependence on others, difficulty in maintaining social contacts, problems in relationships with partners, problems in family life and loss of hobbies. In a number of cases this can lead to depression. The negative impact of rheumatoid arthritis on the physical and psychosocial functioning is one of the causes of the higher degree of sickness absence and employment disability of rheumatoid arthritis patients compared with the Dutch population as a whole (see sections 2.2.2 and 2.2.3).

Rheumatoid arthritis results in an appreciable uptake of health care (i.e. **medical consumption**). Figures for the period 1988-1989 indicate that at least 159,000 GP consultations, at least 140,000 specialist consultations (of which 80-98,000 with a rheumatologist), 4,900 hospital admissions, over 121,000 hospital patient days and at least 360,000 nursing days in nursing homes were attributable (in full or in part) to rheumatoid arthritis.

The figures presented form an *absolute baseline* for the true medical consumption as these are often based on data in which RA was the primary diagnosis. This takes no account of the fact that RA is often the cause of or a contributory factor towards medical consumption without being specifically mentioned in the medical records. The difference can sometimes involve a factor of two to three. On account of lack of data not all centres specifically concerned with rheumatic disorders have been included in the figures. At the risk of stating the obvious, it may be noted that these figures relate only to RA. Had the figures covered all rheumatic diagnosis the numbers would have been much higher (see section 2.2.4).

1.5 Approach selected

Explorations of future developments may be tackled in different ways. One method that has been applied in the Netherlands in recent years is the scenario method.

In a scenario study, a number of possible images of the future are drawn up with the aid of scenarios. A scenario has been defined as follows: "A scenario describes how the present situation for a part of society may be changed into a particular image of the future by means of a series of possible developments. The aim in so doing is to obtain greater insight into the underlying mechanisms and the ways in which these can be influenced" (11).

A distinction is often drawn between exploratory and strategic scenarios. A strategic scenario takes a particular (desired) image of the future and explores the various strategic paths in which this might be achieved. In an exploratory scenario the future is studied by examining a number of differing possible images of the future. This study is based primarily on exploratory scenarios. By drawing a distinction between likely developments on the one hand and possibilities for influencing these developments on the other an attempt has been made to provide a certain structure in the wide range of possibilities inherent in the future.

The steps that any scenario study needs to follow - although not always in the same form, or with the same degree of intensity - are shown in diagrammatic form in Table 1.1

Table 1.1 Stepwise design of a scenario study

Necessary steps	Selected approach in the "Chronic diseases scenario study"
Familiarization with current situation	Background study
Generation of ideas on possible future developments Indication of anticipated effect, degree of probability, point of occurrence, etc. Combination of individual expectations into scenarios	Delphi study followed by workshop
Further elaboration and quantification of scenario effects	Computer model for epidemiology of chronic diseases

Background study

Every scenario study begins with a more or less detailed description of the present situation. This is designed not just to provide insight into possible problems requiring solution but also to identify the factors that will determine future developments. As in the case of diabetes mellitus and CNSLD, a detailed examination has been made in the rheumatoid arthritis scenario study of the available statistical material and the literature, reports and policy documents in relation to both the present scale of the problem and past developments. This background study was completed in November 1990 and provided the basis for Chapter 2 of this report.

Delphi study and workshop

Once the initial situation has been depicted, sets of expectations of future developments may be drawn up. Each set of expectations is based on conjectures concerning possible future developments. An essential feature of these speculative forecasts is that they indicate the anticipated effect, degree of probability and timing, etc. For this purpose the Delphi method is used. Under this method, a systematic survey of future expectations is compiled by means of repeated rounds of questionnaires sent to experts with interim anonymous feedback reports. With respect to the design of the Delphi study, provisional results were available on the background study. With a view to comparability the questionnaire was drawn up in the same way as that for the previously examined disorders, i.e. diabetes mellitus and CNSLD.

While a Delphi study provides the building blocks for future scenarios, these building blocks then need to be combined in an appropriate manner. In order to check for consistency - which forms an indispensable element - a workshop was convened consisting of selected participants in the Delphi study. The Delphi study was conducted between April and October 1990. A draft report was completed by the end of November, which then provided the basis for the workshop in January 1991. The results of the Delphi study and workshop provide the basis for Chapter 3 of this report.

Computer model

At an early stage of the project a start was made on developing various kinds of computer models to trace the impact of demographic trends (i.e. the ageing of the population and growth of the population) on the anticipated number of RA-patients in the period 1990-2005. In this respect it has been assumed that the number of RA-patients per age and sex group remains relatively constant over time. The impact of demographic trends has been examined for two initial levels: one in which the estimate of the number of patients per age and sex group has been derived from epidemiological research and one derived from general practitioners' morbidity records. At an early stage of the project it became clear that, in contrast to diabetes mellitus, the lack of reliable data meant that it was not possible to incorporate changes in the risk of contracting RA and the likelihood of dying from or recovering from RA in a mathematical model. The same applies to CNSLD.

After the scenarios of the future had been elaborated an effort was made to indicate the quantitative effects of the demographic and other potential developments. The results of these calculations are provided in Chapter 4 of this report.

2 CURRENT SITUATION AND BACKGROUND

2.1 Introduction and comments on the concepts employed

The sections below describe the current situation for four aspects of relevance for the compilation of possible scenarios, namely the prevalence of rheumatoid arthritis (RA), the occurrence of articular features and extra-articular manifestations of RA, the quality of life (with particular emphasis on sickness absence and employment disability) and medical consumption. To begin with a survey is provided of the present scale of the problem (section 2.2), after which a comparison is drawn with other countries (section 2.3). In addition past trends are, where possible, examined (section 2.4). Finally, on the basis of past and present data, the main factors of relevance for future developments in this field are outlined (section 2.5).

As noted in Chapter 1, this scenario study is confined to RA as one of the rheumatic disorders. A survey of one of the classifications of rheumatic disorders currently in use is provided in Annex 1 (1). This report does not examine juvenile RA*.

RA is one of the most serious rheumatic disorders, which generally manifests itself after puberty. The disease is characterized by the inflammation of a number of joints (polyarthritis). The cause is unknown. In many cases the disorder is symmetrical, i.e. the same joints are affected in the left and right parts of the body. Although the disorder tends to be concentrated on the small joints of the hands and forefeet, the inflammation can occur in virtually any joint. Pain, stiffness and swelling of the joints are the main features, resulting in loss of function. In the end damage to the joints can lead to serious deformities (i.e. articular features/symptoms) with a marked loss of functional capacity.

A wide range of other features not stemming from the joints may be associated with rheumatoid arthritis (i.e. extra-articular manifestations). While these

---

* Juvenile RA may be said to apply if the inflammation of the joints commences before the age of 16 and four or more joints have been affected over a period of three months. Juvenile chronic arthritis is regarded as a separate disease as it manifests itself differently in both the joints and elsewhere. With a prevalence of 0.2-1.0/1,000 the disorder is also rare in comparison with RA (1).

phenomena are most common in the case of serious forms of rheumatoid arthritis, they may also provide the first symptom of the disorder. Various organs, such as the heart, blood vessels, lungs and kidneys may be involved.

Over the past 35 years the diagnostic (at individual level) and classification (at group level) criteria of RA have been the subject of continual discussion since RA lacks any one specific feature that is always present. The diagnosis/classification of RA involves weighing up a series of indications obtained from case records, physical, serological and radiological research. The highly variable cause of the disorder is a further complicating factor.

In order to permit comparison of the occurrence and course of RA both nationally and internationally, uniform criteria need to be adopted. Diagnostic criteria were first drawn up by the American Rheumatism Association (ARA) in 1956. Following the revision of these criteria in 1958 (3) they have been used worldwide over the past 30 years, especially for classification purposes (Annex 2). These ARA criteria consisted of a list of 11 criteria and 20 exclusions. Depending on the number of criteria satisfied by the patient, a classification was made into classical (seven of the 11 criteria), definite (five of the 11 criteria), probable (three of the 11 criteria, with joint symptoms continuous for at least six weeks) or possible RA (two of the 11 criteria, joint symptoms for at least three months). Subsequently different diagnostic criteria were also developed, such as the Rome criteria of 1961 (4) and the New York criteria of 1966 (5). In 1987 the ARA drew up new classification criteria as developments in the past 30 years had meant that a number of RA clinical pictures could be distinguished and there was an increasing need for the existing ARA criteria to be simplified (Annex 3) (6). The number of criteria has been reduced to seven, of which four are required for classification as RA. The sub-classification into classic, definite, probable and possible has been deleted. The criteria have also been more tightly defined and also place greater demands on clinical skills. These new ARA criteria are those most commonly in use at the present time.

Before describing the present scale of the problem a "model" is shown in Figure 2.1 in order to bring out the interconnections between the occurrence of RA, the occurrence of articular features and extra-articular manifestations of RA, the quality of life and medical consumption. A list of definitions of some of the key concepts used in this report is given in chart 2.1.

Figure 2.1 "Model" illustrating the interrelationships

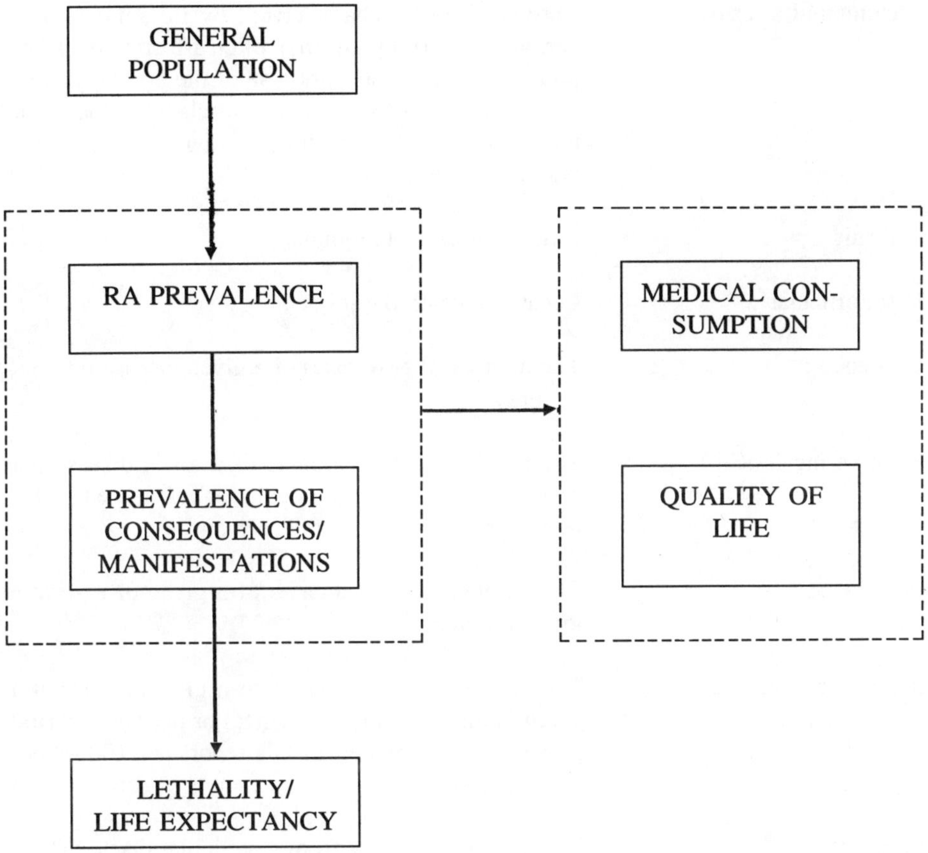

Chart 2.1 Definition of concepts used in this report

Rheumatoid arthritis :	Chronic disorder characterized by inflammation of various joints (polyarthritis), often affecting the same joints in the left and right side of the body (symmetrical). A range of symptoms not related to the joints may also form part of the disorder (extra-articular manifestations).
Arthritis :	Inflammation of the joints.
Extra-articular :	Located outside the joint.
Incidence :	The number of new cases of a given disease per unit of time.
Relative incidence* :	The number of known cases of a given disease per unit of time in a defined population, expressed in this report per 100 or per 1,000 persons.
Prevalence :	The number of known cases of a given disease at a given moment.
Relative prevalence* :	The number of known cases of a given disease at a given moment (point prevalence) or per year (period prevalence), expressed in this report per 100 or per 1,000 persons.
Mortality :	The number of deaths from a particular disease (RA) per unit of time in a defined population, expressed in this report per year and per 100,000.
Lethality :	The risk of dying given the presence of a disease (RA).
Remission :	The chance of temporary or permanent recovery within a given period given the presence of disease (RA).

* Where it is self-evident in the text, the qualification "relative" for the incidence and prevalence has been omitted.

Exacerbation :	Increase in the severity of symptoms and manifestations as a result of active RA.
Consequence/complication :	Condition as a result of RA.
Risk factor :	Factor solely or partly responsible for the onset of a disease, consequence or complication.
Quality of life :	A state of well-being consisting of three components: physical, mental and social functioning.
Medical consumption :	Uptake of health care facilities by RA-patients **as a result of** the disease.

2.2 Current scale of the problem

2.2.1 Occurrence of RA

2.2.1.1 Introduction

The current number of patients with RA (prevalence) is the net result of an inflow and an outflow of patients. The inflow is equal to the incidence; the outflow is the sum of remission and lethality (Figure 2.2).

Figure 2.2 Prevalence of RA as a result of incidence, remission and lethality

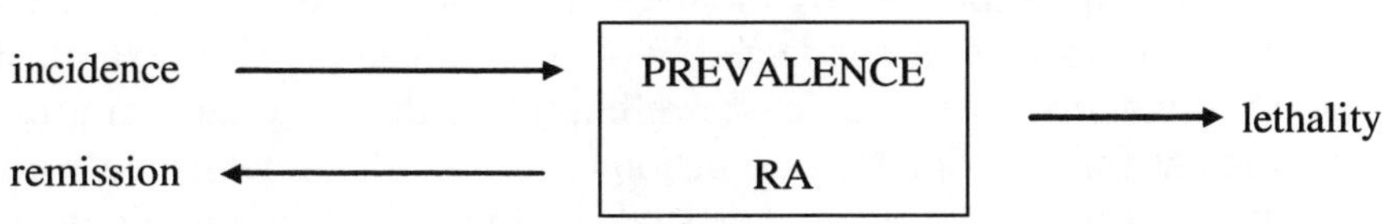

2.2.1.2 Incidence and prevalence

A study of the literature revealed that the *incidence* and/or *prevalence* of RA have been examined in only a few surveys in the Netherlands in the period 1975-1990. In terms of the method of data collection the surveys may be divided into three categories:

1. epidemiological studies.
2. GP morbidity records.
3. questionnaires forming part of population surveys.

The prevalence and incidence data forming the basis for the modelling of future expectations were drawn from the following studies:

1. the **prevalence** of RA among persons aged 20 and over from the Zoetermeer Epidemiological Preventive Survey (EPOZ) (7);
2. the **incidence** and **prevalence** of RA **for all ages** from data from the morbidity records of the Nijmegen University General Practitioners Institute (8).

The various studies are examined in turn, with conclusions on pages 48 and 49.

Prevalence of RA according to epidemiological research
During the period 1975-1978, 3,091 males and 3,493 females aged 20 and over were screened in Zoetermeer for the presence of rheumatological complaints and disorders (prevalence). No information was obtained on the incidence. RA was diagnosed in terms of (i) the old criteria of the American Rheumatism Association (ARA criteria) (3) and (ii) the clinical impression and case records. The diagnosis was made on the basis of the particulars filled in on the questionnaire by the individual concerned and the anamnesis and physical examination conducted by a doctor. The physical examination established whether there was any swelling, disability and pain on pressure or movement for each joint/group of joints. It was also established whether the joint was warmer. No account was taken of the results of radiological and serological tests in assessing the presence of RA. This approach has accordingly been termed the EPOZ diagnosis of RA.

Table 2.1 shows the prevalence of RA by age and sex.

Table 2.1 Prevalence of RA in Zoetermeer by age and sex (EPOZ 1975-1978)

Age	Men		Women	
	%	(n)	%	(n)
20 - 24	0.3	(292)	0.3	(298)
25 - 34	0.0	(662)	0.1	(764)
35 - 44	0.6	(778)	0.1	(833)
45 - 54	0.4	(674)	1.8	(684)
55 - 64	2.0	(398)	3.6	(415)
65 - 74	1.5	(201)	3.0	(305)
75+	1.2	(86)	6.7	(194)

On the basis of the composition of the Dutch population in 1990 and the EPOZ data, the prevalence of RA among those aged 20-75 plus in 1990 amounts to 1.2%. For men and women the figures are 0.7% and 1.8% respectively.

From this it is evident that:

1. standardized in terms of the Dutch population in 1990 aged 20 and over, the prevalence of RA among women was 2.6 times higher than that among men (1.8% and 0.7% respectively).
2. age-specifically the prevalence rises later in life among both men and women, in the case of men after the age of 55 and for women after age 45.
3. age-specifically the prevalence among women aged 45 and over is consistently higher than that among men.

If the occurrence of RA is related not just to the population aged 20 and over but to all ages, the prevalence for men in 1990 was 0.5% and for women 1.3% (with a collective prevalence of 0.9%).

It should be noted that the extent to which these prevalences reflect the true situation is unclear. It is possible that the actual prevalence is underestimated. Factors responsible for such an underestimation include the following. In the first place the possibility of selection bias on account of non-response (approx. 20-40%, depending on age) cannot be ruled out since the non-response group may include a greater number of persons who are not fully mobile, such as RA-patients. Secondly, in making the diagnosis of RA, the EPOZ made no allowance for possible radiological signs and the presence of certain antibodies in the blood (rheumatoid factor). If allowance is made for these factors, the possibility cannot be excluded that RA might have been diagnosed more frequently. Thirdly, individuals who suffered from poly-arthritis in the past have been left out in determining the prevalence of RA, although it is possible that some of these individuals might be enjoying only a temporary remission.

On the other hand the number of individuals covered by the survey in each age and sex group is comparatively small and the data go back some years. It is therefore not inconceivable that the actual prevalence rates in the present Dutch population might differ somewhat. On account of the lack of other, more recent Dutch epidemiological studies, comparison with this study is not possible. A comparison with epidemiological studies in other countries is provided in section 2.3.

It remains notable, however, that in contrast to the situation among women, the prevalence among men fluctuates markedly with age, whereas normally in the case of a chronic disorder it might be expected to rise. Given the comparatively small number of individuals per age group, the possibility that this is due to chance cannot be ruled out. If the fluctuations do reflect reality, the decline in the prevalence among males later in life (from age 65) would need to be explained in terms of the fact that the life expectancy of male RA-patients is more sharply reduced in relation to the male population as a whole than it is among women. The fluctuation of the prevalence among men at younger ages would then need to be explained in terms of remission. The reduction in life expectancy and remission is examined in more detail in section 2.2.1.3.

Table 2.2 shows the absolute number of patients with RA in the Netherlands in 1990, on the assumption that the prevalence figures from the EPOZ survey are representative of the present Dutch population. The numbers have been collapsed into five age categories.

From Table 2.2 it may be seen that:
1. of all RA-patients some 28% are male and 72% female;
2. 72% of male RA-patients are aged under 65, compared with 45% of women (total: 53%);

3. on the basis of the five age groups, the absolute number of patients per age group falls for both men and women from the age of 65. This is due in part to the fall in the number of inhabitants in the Netherlands in the successive age groups.

Table 2.2 Estimated number of patients with RA in the Netherlands in 1990 by age and sex based on an extrapolation of the EPOZ data*

Age	Men	Women	Total
0 - 19	-	-	-
20 - 44	10,497	4,237	14,734
45 - 64	17,287	40,923	58,210
65 - 79	9,227	34,537	43,764
80+	1,617	20,449	22,066
Total	38,628	100,146	138,774

* The prevalences as found in the EPOZ (1975-1978) have been multiplied by the number of inhabitants in the Netherlands in the relevant age and sex category in 1990.

Incidence and prevalence of RA in general practice

There are no epidemiological data from Dutch research on the incidence of RA from 1975 onwards. An old longitudinal epidemiological study conducted in the suburb of Bloemhof in Rotterdam between 1949 and 1963 indicated an annual incidence of 0.87/1000 (9). For more recent data one is dependent on morbidity records from general practice. The Nijmegen University General Practitioners Institute (NUHI) indicates the incidence, expressed in the incidence rate (i.e. the number of new cases/number of person-years) and the number of known cases of RA (including ankylosing spondylitis) in the period 1985-1988 among some 12,000 persons by age and sex (Table 2.3) (8). The disorders have been defined on the basis of the adapted E-list (ICHPPC-2-defined) see Annex 4) (10).

The number of known cases in 1985 has been determined by on-coding the number of new and known cases from 1984, providing the latter remain known as such to their general practitioner. In this way the new (incidence) cases in 1985 only count as known patients in 1986, which is why the number of known patients in 1985 is lower than (and cannot therefore be equated with) the prevalence. When it comes to determining the prevalence, the additional number of new patients each year will in practice add only slightly to the number of new patients in the case of a chronic disease. This may also be seen from Table 2.3, with the exception of the 10-14 years age group. A better approximation of the true prevalence may be obtained by adding half the number of new patients per age group to the number of known patients*. The "prevalence" approximated in this way is shown in the final three columns of Table 2.3. In contrast to the previous tables the relative figures in Table 2.3 are expressed not per 100 persons but per 1,000 person-years.

Table 2.3 **Incidence, number of known cases and "prevalence"* of RA (including ankylosing spondylitis) in the period 1985-1988 by age and sex per 1,000 persons per year (person-years) in the NUHI**

Age	0-4	5-9	10-14	15-24	25-34	35-44	45-54	55-64	65-74	75+
Incidence:										
men	0.0	0.0	1.3	0.0	0.2	0.0	0.8	1.8	2.7	2.4
women	0.0	0.0	0.0	0.0	0.4	0.6	0.0	0.4	1.6	1.4
total	0.0	0.0	0.7	0.0	0.3	0.3	0.4	1.1	2.1	1.8
Known cases:										
men	0.0	0.0	1.3	0.9	2.8	2.2	6.0	8.9	13.5	14.6
women	0.0	0.0	0.0	0.6	1.9	7.9	8.8	10.7	23.5	32.8
total	0.0	0.0	0.7	0.7	2.3	5.0	7.4	9.8	19.0	26.2
"Prevalence":										
men	0.0	0.0	2.0	0.9	2.9	2.2	6.4	9.8	14.9	15.8
women	0.0	0.0	0.0	0.6	2.1	8.2	8.8	10.9	24.3	33.5
total	0.0	0.0	1.1	0.7	2.5	5.2	7.6	10.4	20.1	27.1

* Number of known cases + half the incidence cases

---

* In this respect it is assumed that the incidence patients are on average discovered half way through the year and then contribute towards the prevalence for the remainder of that year.

From Table 2.3 and 2.4 it may be seen that:

1. the ratio between the incidence for the total population and the "prevalence" is 1:12.4 (0.5/1,000 resp. 6.2/1,000);
2. the (relative) "prevalence" for the total population among women is 1.8 times greater than that among men (8.1/1,000 resp. 4.4/1,000), while the incidence among males is 1.5 times greater than that among women (0.6/1,000 resp. 0.4/1,000). This is discussed in greater detail on page 44;
3. age-specifically (for men and women together) the incidence and especially the "prevalence" increases with age;
4. sex-specifically the "prevalence" is greater among men than women up to the age of 35, while from that age onwards the reverse applies. By contrast the incidence is higher for men than women from the age of 45.

On the basis of the composition of the Dutch population in 1990, the NUHI data may be used to calculate the incidence, number of known cases and "prevalence" in 1990. The results are shown in Table 2.4.

Table 2.4 Incidence, number of known cases and "prevalence"* of RA (including ankylosing spondylitis) in 1990 by age per 1,000 persons per year (person-years) in the Netherlands on the basis of NUHI figures

	Incidence	Known cases	"Prevalence"
Men	0.6	4.1	4.4
Women	0.4	7.9	8.1
Total	0.5	6.0	6.2

* Number of known cases + half the incidence cases.

It should be noted that:
1. The age/sex cell size is comparatively small. Caution is therefore in order, particularly when making statements about the incidence, since the latter is 12.4 times smaller than the "prevalence".
2. The "prevalence" refers to the number of RA-patients known to general practitioners. On account of underdiagnosis the true prevalence could well be higher.

3. The incidence and "prevalence" of RA includes ankylosing spondylitis. In relation to RA the latter is, however, comparatively infrequent (prevalence 0.2%, smaller than RA by a factor of 5-10 (11).
4. The number of registered patients below the age of 16 may include patients with juvenile chronic arthritis who fall outside the scope of this scenario study.

It is notable that the prevalence for the total population is 1.8 times greater among women than men, while the incidence among men is 1.5 times greater than among women. Given the comparatively small number of persons in each age group, the possibility that this is due to chance cannot be ruled out. If the figures reflect reality, a higher outflow on account of remission and/or mortality among men would be a possible explanation. There are indications that the life expectancy of male RA-patients is more sharply reduced in relation to the male population as a whole than it is among women. The less marked rise in the prevalence at higher ages among men in relation to women could be the result of this. The reduction in life expectancy and remission is examined in more detail in section 2.2.1.3.

Table 2.5 shows the absolute number of patients with RA in the Netherlands in 1990, on the assumption that the prevalence rates from the NUHI are also representative of the present Dutch population. For the purposes of this survey the figures have been collapsed into five age groups.

Table 2.5 Estimated number of patients with RA (including ankylosing spondylitis) in the Netherlands in 1990 by age and sex on the basis of the NUHI*

Age	Men	Women	Total
0 - 19	1,417	326	1,743
20 - 44	7,066	12,292	19,358
45 - 64	12,337	15,177	27,514
65 - 79	8,820	23,405	32,225
80+	2,879	9,815	12,694
Total	32,519	61,015	93,534

* The prevalences as found in the NUHI (1985-1988) have been multiplied by the number of inhabitants in the Netherlands in the relevant age and sex category in 1990.

Table 2.5 reveals that:

1. Of all RA-patients (including ankylosing spondylitis) approximately 35% are male and 65% are female.
2. 64% of male RA-patients are aged under 65, compared with 46% of female RA-patients (combined 52%).
3. On the basis of the five age categories, the number of male patients per age category rises up to the age of 65, after which it declines. In the case of women the figure rises up to the age of 80 and then falls. The decline in the highest age categories is the result of the fall in the number of inhabitants in those categories, despite the rising prevalence with age (see Table 2.3).
4. Registered patients under the age of 20 account for only 1.9% of the total number of patients. There is therefore only a limited possibility that the true figures are distorted because this category contains patients with juvenile chronic arthritis.

Recent data from surveillance projects in other general practices

In the monograph "General Practice and Chronic Disorders" forming part of the National Study of Diseases and Treatments in General Practice carried out by the NIVEL in 1987-1988, information is also provided on the occurrence of RA in general practice. Provisional analysis suggests that the incidence (0.3/1,000) and prevalence (2.5/1,000) of RA in that specific population is smaller than that recorded by the NUHI (Table 2.3) with a broadly corresponding age and sex-dependent pattern (12). Part of the difference may be explained because the population in the specialized study is comparatively young. Similarly, in a study among persons aged 65 and over in the Groningen region the prevalence is somewhat lower than that according to the NUHI (13). Once again the age and sex-dependent pattern broadly corresponds. Further analysis is required into the causes of these differences.

Comparison of EPOZ and NUHI data

The numbers of patients with RA as recorded in the EPOZ and the NUHI are shown in Tables 2.2 and 2.4 respectively. By way of illustration the absolute numbers of men and women according to the EPOZ and NUHI are shown in graphic form in Figures 2.3 and 2.4.

Figure 2.3 **Estimated number of male patients with RA* in the Netherlands in 1990 by age on the basis of the EPOZ (aged 20 and over) and the NUHI (all ages)****

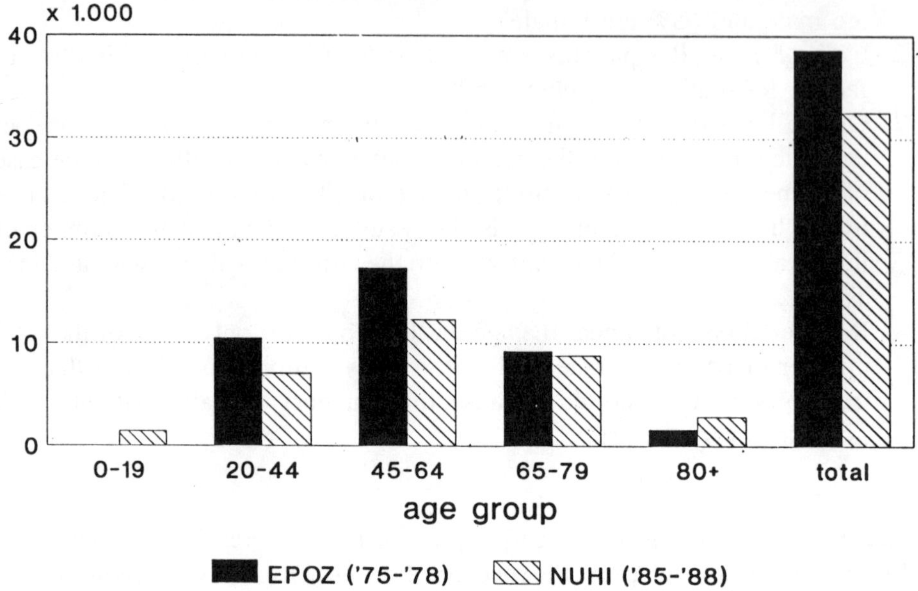

* For the NUHI: including ankylosing spondylitis.

** The prevalences as found in the EPOZ (1975-1978) and NUHI (1985-1988) have been multiplied by the number of inhabitants in the Netherlands in the relevant age and sex groups in 1990.

If the number of patients with RA in the EPOZ is compared with the number as recorded in the NUHI's continuous morbidity surveillance project, the most notable feature is that the number of patients recorded in general practices is significantly lower than that established in the epidemiological study. This applies to both men and women. Age-specifically by sex, however, the picture differs, in that more patients have been recorded in general practice in the 80+ age group for males and the 20-44 age group for females. Those aged under 20 have been left out of account.

The reason for the difference between the number of patients as found in the epidemiological study and that recorded in general practice therefore remains open to conjecture.

Figure 2.4 Estimated number of female patients with RA* in the Netherlands in 1990 by age on the basis of the EPOZ (aged 20 and over) and the NUHI (all ages)**

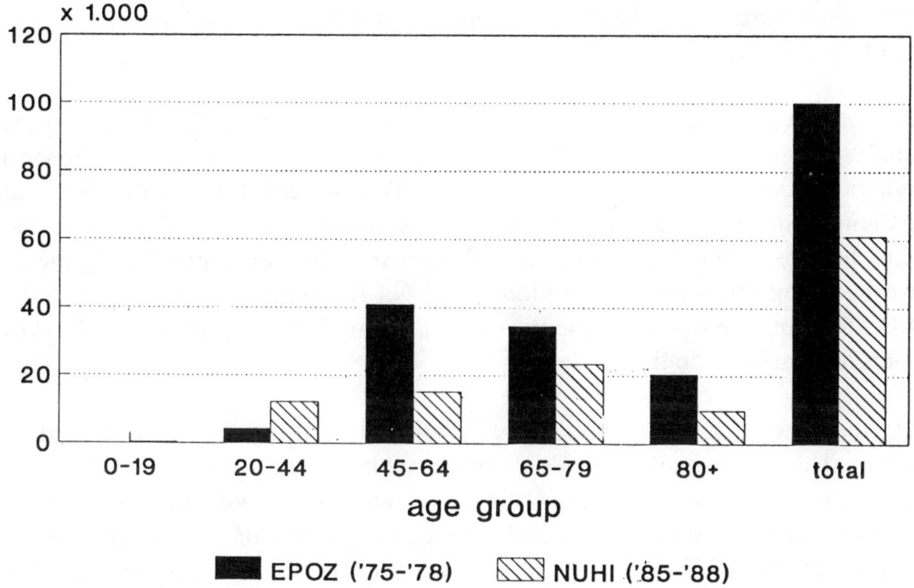

*, **: As for Figure 2.3

The fact that the number of patients according to the epidemiological study (with the exception of the 80+ age group for men and the 20-44 age group for women) is larger than that according to the general practice records may be attributable to:

1. Differences in diagnostic criteria;
2. Underdiagnosis in general practice. This could apply especially to less serious forms of the disease.
3. Underreporting in general practice. This depends on the quality of the records, i.e. the scrupulousness with which the doctor records patients diagnosed as having RA.
4. The differing periods in which the surveys were conducted. On the assumption that the surveys were conducted on much the same basis, this would then indicate a decline in the prevalence over time.

The reason why the number of patients in the 80+ age group for men and the 20-44 age group for women should be greater in the general practice records than in the epidemiological study is unclear. A plausible explanation might be that general practitioners detect cases with a highly variable course at an earlier stage; the epidemiological study is, after all, a snapshot in time. Why this should be confined to these age groups is unclear. Nor is it clear whether the non-response in these age groups generated a selection bias in the epidemiological study.

Matters are, however, even more complicated. Within the EPOZ a separate analysis was carried out by comparing the "epidemiological" and the "general practice" diagnoses at individual level. This revealed that only 60% of patients who reported that they were being treated by their GP for RA had this diagnosis confirmed in the EPOZ. GPs therefore evidently treat patients for RA even though these individuals are not RA-patients accordingly to the EPOZ. It may be that this largely concerns individuals in whom the RA takes a highly variable course.

On the other hand, the analysis revealed that of the patients diagnosed as having RA according to the EPOZ, approximately *three-quarters* had at some point consulted their GP concerning problems to do with their musculoskeletal system. It also turned out that at least *a quarter of these patients* were known by their GPs to have RA. According to the EPOZ, therefore, the percentage of RA-patients recorded as such by their GP is in the range of 20-75%.

Conclusion

The age and sex-specific prevalences of RA as established by the epidemiological study and general practice records differ considerably. As a basis for modelling future expectations with respect to the number of RA-patients, both the EPOZ and the NUHI data will therefore be used. The epidemiological study provides an insight into the prevalence of RA in the population, whereas the continuous morbidity registration provides an insight into the occurrence of RA cases known to the medical profession.

This distinction is necessary for calculating the medical consumption as a result of RA. On the one hand the medical consumption related to the prevalence of RA according to the morbidity registration figures will probably be an underestimate since the epidemiological study suggests that it is quite possible that RA-patients could make use of medical facilities on account of their RA without being diagnosed as such by their GP. On the other hand, a decision to equate the medical consumption of RA-patients who are not known to their general practitioner with the medical consumption of

RA-patients who have been diagnosed as such by their general practitioner would probably lead to an overestimate of the total medical consumption, on the grounds that the additional RA-patients detected by the epidemiological study might have a less serious form of RA and therefore draw less heavily on medical facilities.

2.2.1.3 Remission and lethality

There are few data on the contribution of complete and lasting *remission* (i.e. recovery) to the outflow from the RA population (see Figure 2.2). Most surveys are concerned with mortality (i.e. life expectancy) as the final outcome of RA, while little attention is devoted to the course of the disease. On the basis of various surveys it is generally assumed that some 20% of patients in specialist care enjoy a complete remission, while 50% have a slow progressive form of RA. With respect to the latter form, it needs to be borne in mind that it can in due course also result in joint deformity (personal communication by Van Rijswijk, Groningen). Chronic active RA with progressive damage to the joints, frequently accompanied by extra-articular manifestations, occurs in 25% of cases, while 5% develop progressive, serious RA (14-16).

Caution is however in order when it comes to interpretation. On the one hand there is a certain degree of selection bias, since the survey only covers patients being treated by specialists. The results could therefore form a negative reflection of the true state of affairs, in that patients with less serious forms of RA have been left out of account. In addition the surveys are not of recent date, so that it is not inconceivable that the likelihood of remission will have improved with the introduction of new forms of medical treatment.

On the other hand it is also possible that the situation is viewed overoptimistically. In the first place, the description of the course of RA is confined to patients who are still alive, thus introducing a selection bias. In a 20-year follow-up survey it turned out that among the RA-patients who had died before the end of the 20-year period, 35% were ultimately confined to a wheelchair or bed (Steinbrocker grade IV) (see section 2.2.3) and 24% were severely limited in daily activities (Steinbröcker grade III) (17). Secondly, these surveys could cover patients who were diagnosed at the time as having RA but who would no longer be diagnosed as such in terms of the present criteria. It is therefore conceivable that less serious non-RA-patients were included in the study as RA-patients. There is no recent longitudinal study into the prognosis for the total (unselected) group of RA-patients according to current criteria (i.e. a research blank spot).

Apart from cases of complete remission, the outflow from the RA population is determined by *lethality*. In the Netherlands we have the cause-of-death statistics of the Central Bureau of Statistics (CBS). On the basis of the International Classification of Diseases (ICD) both the underlying cause of death (i.e. primary cause of death) and other diseases that were a contributory factor towards the death (i.e. secondary causes of death) are recorded. The primary and secondary causes of death for RA (code 714) do not provide a direct insight into the lethality among RA-patients but can be used to throw some light on the subject.

Table 2.6 shows mortality from RA as the primary and secondary cause of death (code 714) by age and sex in 1988 (18). The table reveals that:

1. Some 6 persons per 100,000 inhabitants die each year with RA as the (primary or secondary) cause of death. Converted this corresponds to some 880 deaths in the Netherlands per year. Of these RA is the primary cause of death in around 37% of cases and the secondary cause of death in some 63% of cases (not included in the table);
2. The total mortality with RA as the (primary or secondary) cause of death per 100,000 is 2.4 times higher for women than for men. This is in the same order of magnitude as that calculated for prevalence (2.6 according to the EPOZ; 1.8 according to the NUHI);
3. Age-specifically the mortality with RA as (primary or secondary) cause of death per 100,000 inhabitants rises sharply with age, especially in the case of women.

If the primary and secondary causes of death are aggregated, RA accounted in 1988 for 0.4% of the total number of deaths among males and 1.1% among females. For both sexes the figure comes to 0.7%.

Caution is however in order when it comes to interpreting these figures. The percentages shown are presumably much lower than the true state of affairs. In the first place the Dutch cause-of-death certificates are wholly directed towards obtaining information concerning indications of the primary cause of death. Secondly, multiple pathology can - especially at later ages - lead to the underregistration of chronic diseases (including RA) as the secondary cause of death. The fact that RA is not specified on the death certificate even though many individuals suffered from serious and incapacitating RA emerges from a Swedish study (19). Of 84 deceased RA-patients, RA was shown on the death certificate in only nine cases (approx. 11%), of which four as primary and five as the secondary cause of death. A corresponding (unpublished) survey in Rotterdam in 1975 came up with a figure of 10% for the Netherlands (personal communication by Valkenburg, Amsterdam).

Table 2.6 Mortality of RA-patients* per 100,000 inhabitants (and absolute), by age and sex in 1988 (CBS)

Sex	Age group (years)					
	0-19	20-44	45-64	65-79	80+	Total
Men	0.0 (0)	<1.0 (2)	3.5 (52)	23.4 (142)	47.5 (61)	3.5 (257)
Women	0.0 (0)	0.0 (0)	3.0 (45)	32.1 (266)	112.9 (313)	8.4 (624)
Total	0.0 (0)	<1.0 (2)	3.2 (97)	28.5 (408)	92.2 (374)	6.0 (881)

* Primary and secondary causes of death for mortality from RA (code 714)

Another method for determining the outflow from the RA population as a result of lethality is by making use of data on the reduction in life-expectancy among RA-patients in relation to the population as a whole. This method was applied in the scenario report on diabetes mellitus (20). Extensive research has been conducted into the life expectancy of RA-patients (e.g. 17, 19, 21-31). With one exception (27) it may be concluded on the basis of these surveys that RA-patients suffer from a reduction in life-expectancy in relation to the population in general. Differences in the survey methods (e.g. differences in diagnostic criteria, patient selection (hospital, open population) and in the length of the follow-up period) make it impossible to express that reduction in years. A Dutch survey with the longest follow-up period of 25 years (29) indicated that the median life-expectancy (i.e. the point at which 50% of the individuals have died) was seven years shorter for men and three years shorter for women with RA compared with the general population. The survey related to RA-patients being treated by a specialist.

A number of the surveys referred to above suggest that the reduction in life-expectancy is not the same for all RA-patients, being particularly pronounced among patients suffering from a serious form of RA at an early stage of the disease. A survey conducted by Rasker and Cosh (17) showed that 46 out of 100 RA-patients had died in a 20-year follow-up period. Of these nine had died some 15 years earlier than expected as a result of RA or extra-articular manifestations, while eight patients among whom RA was a contributory cause of death died 10 years earlier than expected. Among the 29 patients whose death could not be related to RA, the age at death was five years earlier than might otherwise have been expected.

The extent to which the reduction in life-expectancy associated with serious forms of RA early on in the course of the disease is due to a functional immunodeficiency or other genetically determined factors and the extent to which it is attributable to intoxications from drugs used in the treatment of serious forms of RA is not known with any certainty (32). Prospective epidemiological research into the mortality from RA in which the immune function and heredity (HLA-type) are included at an early stage of the disease should be encouraged with a view to assessing its predictive significance (32). Among other things this would make it possible to gear the therapeutic plan to the underlying process (research blank spot).

Conclusion

On account of the lack of usable adequate data concerning the outflow from the RA population on the one hand (as a result of remission and lethality/-reduction in life-expectancy) and the inflow on the other (incidence, see section 2.2.1.2), the projections are necessarily based on a static or equilibrium model (see section 4.2.1). This model assumes that in age and sex-specific terms the inflow of new patients is equal to the outflow of known patients. It is consequently assumed that the age and sex-specific prevalences remain constant over time. This is in line with experts' expectations (see Chapter 3).

2.2.1.4 Risk factors

The cause of RA remains the subject of considerable uncertainty. It is assumed that exposure to **primary causative agents** (antigens) of individuals with an **immunogenetic predisposition** can result in the onset of rheumatoid arthritis. This is associated with an abnormal reaction of the immune system, which plays a central role in the onset and progression of articular and extra-articular disorders that are characteristic of rheumatoid arthritis.

Immunogenetic predisposition

It has been demonstrated that the prevalence of RA is six times as high among first-degree family members of a person with a sero-positive form of RA than among controls, while among identical twins the prevalence is over 30 times as high (33). These figures point strongly in the direction of a polygenetic pattern of inheritance. These results are supported by surveys showing an association between RA and the presence of genetically determined antigens (HLA-DR4 and HLA-DR1) in body cells playing a role in the immune system (34-38). Dutch research reveals no significant difference between the occurrence of HLA-DR4 among RA-patients in a population survey (c. 30%) compared with controls (25%) (39). By contrast 60-70% of the RA-patients found in clinical surveys are HLA-DR4 positive, with the figure rising to as much as 90% for RA-patients also suffering from extra-articular manifestations (vasculitis, Felty's syndrome: see section 2.2) (40). There is evidently a genetic heterogeneity within RA (41). These figures also correspond with international research findings (42-44).

Primary aetiologic agents (antigens)

The agents responsible for the onset of RA among persons with an immunogenetic predisposition are unknown. Current research focuses on *exogenous infectious agents* and *endogenous agents*. It is however possible that many other aetiologic agents play a role.

Various viruses (including Ebstein-Barr and parvoviruses) and bacteria (e.g. mycobacteria) have been cited as exogenous infectious agents (45, 46). It has not, however, so far been demonstrated that these infectious agents can in fact be held primarily responsible for the onset of RA.

There is little doubt that auto-immunity is a significant factor in the progression of RA. The evidence is, however, less persuasive that auto-immunity may be regarded as the primary cause of RA. In this respect the main endogenous agents cited are synovial membrane proteins (collagen, proteoglycans) and immunoglobulins (Ig-G) (47).

It is a generally accepted fact that the prevalence of definite RA (see Annex 2) rises with **age** for both men and women (48). The occurrence of RA is notably **sex-related**; the disease is 2-3 times more frequent among women. In those cases where the disease manifests itself before the age of 60, RA is encountered at least five times more frequently among women and twice or less after that age (48-51). The decline in the ratio after the age of 60 may be the result of an abrupt rise in RA among older men (49). The fact that RA is particularly frequent among young women suggests that **hormonal factors** play a role.

A recent dissertation in the Netherlands discusses the use of oral contraceptives (the "pill") in relation to RA (52). This provides once more supportive evidence that the pill has a preventive effect on the onset of RA. The conflicting results in the literature concerning the pill and RA could possibly be explained by shortcomings in the methodology. The method of patient selection is particularly important in this respect; in a number of studies preventive effects can be established for patients being treated by specialists but not for patients drawn from the general population. The signs are therefore that the pill only reduces the risk of RA among a specific subgroup of RA-patients among whom the disease takes a serious course. A recent study, however, suggests that the pill may prevent the disease from becoming seriously progressive (53). A number of studies also suggest that reproduction has a preventive effect on the onset of RA (52, 54, 55).

There is as yet no plausible biological explanation for the influence of the pill and pregnancy on the occurrence or course of RA. The extent to which this is due to the impact of sex hormones on the immune system requires further investigation.

In addition there are indications that RA is more frequent among single householders and divorced women (56) and among persons on lower incomes and with a lower level of education (57). The geographical distribution of RA is examined separately in section 2.3.

Conclusion

The pathogenesis of RA is a complex whole in which various factors are involved. The disease is caused by unidentified agents among persons with an immunogenetic predisposition. An abnormal reaction of the immune system is a key factor. In combination these factors may be held responsible for the deformation of the joints and possible damage to other (extra-articular) organs. Much remains unclear and requires further research.

2.2.2 Articular features and extra-articular manifestations of RA

2.2.2.1 Introduction

RA is a systemic disease, the most characteristic feature of which is the occurrence of inflammation in various joints. In most cases the features are not confined to the joints but one or more other organs or organ systems may display symptoms or abnormalities. In some cases these may be life-threatening and more significant that the articular symptoms.

There are various ways of classifying the features associated with RA. For the purposes of this report a distinction has been drawn between features of RA associated with the joints (i.e. articular features) and those that manifest themselves outside the joints (extra-articular manifestations). The final part of this section is devoted to iatrogenic complications, i.e. complications that are not a direct result of the disease itself but of the treatment. For ease of reference the articular features and extra-articular manifestations of most importance in terms of occurrence and severity are shown in chart 2.2.

This section does not discuss loss of appetite or weight, fever, Raynaud's phenomenon, blood-count disorders, certain heart disorders, disorders of the gastro-intestinal system, liver, eyes and kidneys, other than on the basis of amyloidosis. These extra-articular manifestations are less frequent, less serious or demand less care.

Since the direct cause is not evident for most articular features and extra-articular manifestations this aspect will not be pursued further. The aim of this section is to provide a survey of the complaints associated with the symptoms of RA, the burden these impose on the patient and, where possible, how frequently the symptoms occur. The latter has been done partly so as to provide an indication of the demand for care.

This section is largely based on foreign literature as there is little Dutch literature in this field.

Chart 2.2 Classification of articular features, extra-articular manifestations and iatrogenic complications of RA

Articular features
- pain in the joints
- morning stiffness
- soft-tissue swelling
- loss of function
- deformity

Extra-articular manifestations
- anaemia, chronic fatigue
- osteoporosis and fractures
- peripheral neuropathy
- cervical myelopathy
- subcutaneous nodules
- Sjögren's syndrome
- vasculitis
- lung disorders
- Felty's syndrome
- secondary amyloidosis
- septic arthritis

Iatrogenic complications
as a result of:
- non-steroidal anti-inflammatory drugs (NSAIDs)
- disease-modifying anti-rheumatic drugs (DMARDs)
- corticosteroids
- chemical/radiological synovectomy
- surgery

2.2.2.2 Articular features

Pain in the joints

One of the dominant symptoms in the early stages of the disease is pain. In many cases the pain is most prominent in the morning (58). There may also be discomfort on resting, and in some cases only on moving the joint (59). The pain is affected by external conditions, such as cold and damp (58). In many cases the pain is at its most intense in the earliest stage of the disease, later generally declining in intensity as the rheumatic process is brought to rest by the prescribed treatment (60).

A survey in the Netherlands covering 6,585 people in the open population identified 73 RA-patients, of whom nearly 60% had pain in the joints, compared with 34% in the total population aged 20 and over. More women than men reported pain (7).

A study by McKenna and Wright revealed that RA-patients regard pain as the most important symptom (61). Another survey found that discomfort was the most important motive for seeking medical treatment among roughly 50% of the RA-patients (62). A survey conducted among retired members of the armed forces with RA indicated a strong link between psychological variables (stress) and income on the one hand and pain on the other (63).

Another Dutch study conducted by Rasker et al. among 203 RA-patients drawn at random by sex and degree of urbanization of their place of residence from the database of a rheumatology centre indicated that many patients suffered from pain in the joints. Roughly a quarter of the respondents proved to suffer pain from time to time in each of the joints investigated while some 40% suffered frequent pain. Pain is a factor for all patients. For 38% of the respondents it is one of the biggest problems of the disease, and for a quarter the biggest problem. Pain is closely related to dependence on others (64).

Morning stiffness

A striking complaint of RA, including at an early stage, is generalized morning stiffness throughout the body. The duration and intensity vary with the activity of the inflammation process. In some cases the morning stiffness can last for several hours. Generally it eases with movement. The stiffness is closely related to external factors, such as cold and damp.

The study conducted in the Netherlands by Rasker (see above) showed that many patients regularly suffered from stiff joints. For each of the joints investigated roughly 40% of the respondents suffered frequent stiffness and some 20% occasional stiffness. The figures for the fingers, hands, wrists and feet were somewhat higher than those for the neck, shoulders, elbows and knees. For 15% of the respondents stiffness is one of the major problems of the disease and for 7% the biggest problem of all (64).

Soft-tissue swelling
In the early stage of the disease the swelling of the joints, especially the hands and feet, is one of the dominant symptoms. Swelling in a joint can affect nearby tissue. If this should happen to be nerves, this can result in neurological compression syndrome, with (for example) pain in the fingers or neck and back of the head (see peripheral neuropathy). At the same time the tendon sheaths, tendons and mucous membranes can display the same inflammation symptoms, including swelling, as the joints (58).

Loss of function
Loss of function may occur in any joint and is caused by stiffness, pain, muscular spasms (65) and destruction of the joint (59). The synovial membrane of ligaments and sockets also plays a part. The wastage of muscle tissue and tendon disorders can cause further aggravation (66), until the joints finally stiffen up entirely (ankylosis).

Deformities
Joint deformities generally indicate a protracted, serious disease progression. Various forms are associated with RA, such as partial and total dislocation, instability, displacement and muscle compression (58). Deformities of the fingers are characteristic changes. Knee disorders are the most common reasons for needing a wheelchair (67).

Rasker's survey indicated that for each of the joints investigated a certain percentage of patients suffer from deformities. The percentages vary from 7% (neck) to 34-41% (wrists, feet, hands and fingers) (64).

2.2.2.3 Extra-articular manifestations

Anaemia/chronic fatigue
Anaemia means that the number of red blood cells and/or the haemoglobin count in the blood is lower than normal. The most important complaints caused by anaemia are general malaise, fatigue, weakness, paleness, palpitations, shortness of breath upon exertion, headaches, dizziness and noises in the ear (68).

Anaemia forms part of the RA clinical picture. Apart from abnormalities in the production and storage of red blood cells, anaemia can result from a loss of blood in the gastro-intestinal system on account of the use of anti-rheumatic drugs, but this cause of anaemia is not particularly frequent (69). Intra-articular blood loss can also be a factor (70). Other forms of anaemia are less common (71). The degree of anaemia corresponds with the activity of the disease (69).

RA is almost always associated with some form of anaemia (71, 69). Some two-thirds of the patients examined early in the disease process suffered from mild anaemia (72).

Roughly 30% complain of fatigue (73). For 20% of the respondents fatigue is one of the biggest problems of the disease, and for 11% the biggest problem of all (64).

Osteoporosis and fractures

Osteoporosis is a skeletal disorder in which the quantity of bone tissue is reduced. When the skeleton is no longer able to provide sufficient support, minor injuries can lead to fractures (68), particularly among patients with joint replacements (74). Osteoporosis around the joint may be detected by X-ray at an early stage of the disease process (75).

Osteoporosis also occurs in sites distant from joints, especially in the case of serious and long-standing RA. Risk factors particularly associated with RA-patients are old age, female sex (women in the menopause) immobility, poor posture and movement, poor diet, excessive protein breakdown and the use of corticosteroids (76).

Peripheral neuropathy

Peripheral neuropathy (a disorder of the peripheral nerves) may be subdivided into compression neuropathy and polyneuropathy. *Compression neuropathy* or neurological compression syndrome arises because the swollen tissue around the joints presses against peripheral nerves. The severity of the neurological symptoms depends on the disease-activity of the joint in question. Both exacerbations and remissions may occur. In most cases both motor function (i.e. muscle movement) and sensation are disturbed. Treatment with medicines or operations can greatly alleviate the complaints. Of all the compression neuropathies the most common is compression of the median nerve in the wrist. This results in carpal tunnel syndrome, with a loss of sensation, tingling and pain in the fingers, atrophy of the ball of the thumb and reduced mobility of the thumb. This can occur at any stage of RA (77).

Polyneuropathy (a disturbance of a number of nerves at once) is almost always the result of an inflammation of the connective tissue or the blood vessels surrounding the nerves. Depending on the affected nerves, disturbance may be caused to the motor function (i.e. reduced muscle-power) and to sensory function (i.e. reduced sensation or a burning feeling). In serious cases polyneuropathy can lead to severe disability and death.

Peripheral neuropathy is the most common neurological disorder in RA (77). According to Barnes it is encountered among 33% of patients with serious rheumatoid-factor-positive RA (71). According to Hamburger, however, as many as 45% of patients with chronic RA are estimated to suffer from *compression neuropathy* (78). In the long term two-thirds of RA-patients develop *carpal tunnel syndrome* (71). Among patients with long-standing RA, a more or less serious form of *polyneuropathy* is common after the passage of time (78). In a survey among hospitalized RA-patients, published in 1947, a rate of 84% was encountered (77). Polyneuropathy with disturbances in sensation is the most common form of this disorder (77).

Cervical myelopathy

In the case of serious RA the cervical vertebra are often affected, especially the upper ones. Partial dislocation of these vertebrae can result in narrowing of the spinal canal upon bending the neck, thereby generating pressure on the spinal cord. Symptoms include involuntary movements of the legs, headache, changes in consciousness, loss of sphincter control resulting in incontinence, tingling or numbness in the hands and feet, dizziness and muscular weakness. In many cases, however, there are no complaints at all. In due course the dislocation can result in serious paralysis. In some cases the symptoms arise as a result of the (partial) compression of the spinal-column artery (77), but this is rare (79).

Cervical myelopathy generally arises only late in the progression of the disease in an already seriously disabled patient. In these cases the symptoms are not immediately noticeable (58).

According to Van Soesbergen and Hamburger, figures in the literature on the occurrence of disorders of the cervical vertebrae range from 25% to 90% of RA-patients (79). This depends on the way in which the disorders are defined. Partial dislocation of the upper cervical vertebrae are encountered among some 25% of serious RA-patients (77, 69). Fewer than 10% of patients with a large, radiologically determined dislocation of the cervical vertebrae ultimately develop neurological symptoms attributable to pressure on the spinal cord or (partial) compression of the spinal column artery (69).

Subcutaneous nodules

Subcutaneous nodules are the most specific clinical feature of RA. They are particularly common on the extensor surface of the elbow. They may also occur on the extensor surface of the finger joints, above the kneecap and sometimes on the toes. Sporadically they may also occur elsewhere (58). The subcutaneous nodules are painless (67).

Repeated pressure is probably a factor in the origin and position of subcutaneous nodules. The size of the nodules may vary from less than a millimetre to several centimetres. In most cases they are located below the skin but in some cases they arise from a bursa, tendon, tendon sheath or periosteum and they may also be found in various organs, including the heart, lungs, brains, eyes and kidneys.

Occasionally the nodules can change form, become infected or atrophy (58). In these circumstances the nodules can start to form ulcers. This tends to be painful and is slow-healing (69). Apart from cases of infection and cosmetic aspects, nodules rarely cause problems (71).

Subcutaneous nodules are encountered among roughly 15-30% of patients with definitive or classic RA (annex 2) (59, 58, 65, 73). Prevalence rates of as high as 70% are, however, also encountered (73).

Sjögren's syndrome

RA-patients suffering from keratoconjunctivitis sicca and xerostomia are said to have Sjögren's syndrome. Keratoconjunctivitis sicca is an inflammation of the conjunctiva (i.e. the connective tissue covering the eyeball), the cornea and the tear glands. It is associated with itchiness and a burning feeling in the eyes, loss of visual acuity and reduced secretion of tears. In serious cases keratoconjunctivitis can give rise to scleritis (i.e. inflammation of the white, hard sclera). This is a painful disorder associated with red eyes and reduced visual acuity (58). Xerostomia is a disorder in which the salivary glands are inflamed, leading to dryness of the mouth. Female patients also often suffer from a dry vagina. They are often very reluctant to speak about this, which can have major psychosocial consequences.

Treatment is limited to good oral and eye hygiene, the application of artificial tears and rinsing the mouth with glycerin.

Careful diagnosis indicates that Sjögren's syndrome occurs among some 25% of RA-patients. The existence of the syndrome also entails an increased risk of other extra-articular complications such as vasculitis and Felty's syndrome (58). On the other hand it has also been reported that the prevalence of keratoconjunctivitis sicca among patients with definite RA is over 10%, while the prevalence of scleritis as established in surveys ranges from less than 1% (80) to over 5% of RA-patients (58).

Vasculitis

Vasculitis is an inflammation of the walls of blood vessels. The most prevalent form tends to be encountered in the small arteries, such as those of the fingers and toes. The gangrene resulting from vasculitis can give rise to typical black spots on the fingertips and cuticles known as *digital vasculitis*. Although rarely serious it can sometimes result in gangrene of a finger or toe.

Where the major arteries are attacked vasculitis can be a life-threatening complication (81). The clinical picture of *generalized vasculitis* depends on the size and location of the arteries affected. It also depends on whether the inflammation leads to a fissure, narrowing or widening of the lining of the vessels (67). The condition may give rise to leg ulcers, which can be very hard to clear up. Closure of the blood vessels supplying the nerves with blood results in peripheral neuropathy (see neurological disorders) (67). Generalized vasculitis can also lead to infarcts in, for example, the heart, skeletal muscles and the small intestine (58, 82).

Vasculitis is probably at the heart of numerous extra-articular symptoms. Although the precise cause is unknown, one factor could be the deposition of immunoglobulins in blood-vessel walls (82).

Vasculitis is thought to be of some significance among the majority of RA-patients (65, 58), especially those with subcutaneous nodules and who have tested positively for the rheumatoid factor (59). Autopsies conducted on deceased RA-patients indicate vasculitis in over 25% of cases (69). Definite digital vasculitis, however, is encountered among only 8% of hospitalized patients. Serious generalized vasculitis (with for example neuropathy and gangrene of the fingers) is nowadays diagnosed only rarely. The prevalence detected by various researchers ranges from 0% to 3% (69, 81). A group of

RA-patients with generalized vasculitis were found to have a 5-year life-expectancy of 70% (82).

Pulmonary disorders

Respiratory infections are the most common lung disorder among RA-patients. This is explained by their reduced resistance (82). Possible other risk factors for the development of respiratory infections are reduced pulmonary function (on account of changes in the blood vessels), muscular weakness and disability (69).

Pleurisy (inflammation of the membrane lining the chest cavity) is more common among RA-patients. The most common is the exudative form, in which inflammation fluid is formed. Generally this disorder takes a benign course among RA-patients, although it can remain in evidence for years (58) and can lead to difficulty in breathing, pain (82) and the formation of pus.

There is evidence that *diffuse pulmonary fibrosis* is more common among RA-patients than healthy individuals, especially among rheumatoid factor-positive patients (71). The condition results in a build-up of connective tissue in the lungs. The extent to which it is in fact related to RA remains open to question (83, 69); it may be that it is simply a type of pulmonary fibrosis that occurs more frequently among RA-patients (84). Pulmonary fibrosis may result from the side-effects of medication (e.g. gold and methotrexate). Clinical features include shortness of breath on exertion, coughing and pleuritic pain. In the progressive form the complaints can become extremely serious and even lead to death. Spontaneous remission is very rare (85). In some cases there are no symptoms and the disorder is confined to radiological or pulmonary function abnormalities (82). A specific feature of RA is the occurrence of *granuloma* (rheumatoid nodules) in the lungs. This is however extremely rare (58, 83).

Among patients with only minor deformities of the joints and who are rheumatoid factor negative, the incidence of respiratory disorders is around 1%, rising to approximately 70% among patients with serious joint involvements and patientswhich are strongly seropositive. In some cases the lung disorders can precede the joint involvements by several years. Apart from simple respiratory infections, disorders of the pleura are probably the most common lung disorder in RA (82), occurring amount 50% of RA-patients (86).

The frequency of *exudative pleurisy* as cited in the literature tends to vary, from 0.6% (84) to around 50% (58). It is said to occur particulary among men (58). A prevalence of around 20% has been found for pleurisy without the formation of a pleural effusion; this compares with 10% among a control group of hospital patients (84).

Diffuse pulmonary fibrosis is detected by X-ray diagnosis among roughly 1.6%-11% of RA-patients (83, 84, 85). X-rays tend, however, to be a fairly inaccurate means of detecting pulmonary dysfunction (87). According to Roschmann approximately 30-40% of RA-patients display radiological abnormalities or suffer from abnormal lung function deriving from pulmonary fibrosis or a lung disease (85).

A *rheumatoid nodule* is a comparatively infrequent pulmonary manifestation of RA. Jurik detected a prevalence of 0.3% (84). Where it occurs, this is generally at an advanced stage of RA (82).

Felty's syndrome

Felty's syndrome describes the combination of RA, enlargement of the spleen (splenomegaly) and reduction of the number of white blood cells (leukopenia). The size of the spleen can vary considerably (58). Splenomegaly and leukopenia can flare up independently of one another and go into remission (69). In many cases there is swelling of the lymph glands and the liver. Approximately a quarter of the patients have a notably grey pigmentation in the region of the joints of the extremities and sometimes the face. Not infrequently the patients with this syndrome suffer from other complications.

The leukopenia can be marked (i.e. a very low white blood-cell count. This can give rise to infections; leg ulcers are for example common in patients with Felty's syndrome. In many cases there is also a moderate to sharp reduction in the number of blood platelets, and in some cases anaemia.

Felty's syndrome is diagnosed in 0.5-1% of RA-patients. Generally speaking these are patients with a classical RA (see annex 2) (58), with a demonstrable rheumatoid factor in the blood (71). According to Decker it is encountered among fewer than 5% of the RA-patients who seek medical aid (69).

Felty's syndrome seldom arises in the early stages of rheumatoid disease; more commonly it occurs after some 10 or 20 years. Generally there are also deformities of the joints (58). The course of the disease tends to vary and be unpredictable. Now and then there are cases of spontaneous remission (71). Roughly half the patients have an increased susceptibility to bacterial infections (58). A survey conducted among 27 RA-patients with Felty's syndrome revealed that 41% had chronic leg ulcers and 52% bacterial infections (69).

Secondary amyloidosis

Amyloidosis is the leading cause of kidney disorders in RA. It involves the deposition of a dense, insoluble material (amyloid) in the kidney (88). Amyloid may also be deposited in other organs, such as the gastro-intestinal system, the liver, the heart and the glands, but the kidneys are the most commonly affected (89). The first symptom to show up is loss of protein in the urine (proteinuria), leading to a build-up of fluid in the tissues (oedema). In due course it can give rise to serious renal impairment (59).

The occurrence of amyloidosis is closely related to the duration (71), severity and progression of RA (58). The clinical features emerge at the earliest five years after the onset of RA (58), but on average only after 16 years (89). Whether proper control and medication in RA can influence the onset and cause of amyloidosis remains unclear (71, 89, 58, 88).

It is difficult to provide a prevalence rate for this complication as this depends heavily on the method of research (58, 88). No sound epidemiological research is available (89).
A number of researchers have attempted to arrive at an estimate of the percentage of RA-patients suffering from amyloidosis by means of autopsies on deceased RA-patients. The results of these studies range from roughly 15% to 60% (58, 59, 67, 71, 89).

Clinical features (confirmed by biopsy) are encountered among 5-11% of serious RA-patients (58, 88). Men with RA have a greater chance of developing amyloidosis than women with RA (89).

In a longitudinal study among 1,000 RA-patients and 1,000 controls, 352 RA-patients and 217 controls had died at the end of a follow-up period of 10 years. Of the deceased RA-patients 8.8% had died as a result of amyloidosis and 11.9% as a result of other renal impairment. Of the deceased controls the percentages for both causes of death were 0.5% (90).

Septic arthritis

Septic arthritis is a serious complication (67, 71). In this condition micro-organisms (bacteria) infiltrate from the bloodstream into one or more joints or into various organs (76). As a result of the condition, acute symptoms can suddenly flare up in an affected joint. In serious cases the septic arthritis is associated with high fever and swollen, hot and very painful joints. Generally only one joint is affected, but it is also common for several joints to be affected. It is often difficult to distinguish septic arthritis from RA itself. Sometimes septic arthritis is therefore not recognized as such, as the symptoms also occur in uncomplicated RA. In 50% of cases there may even be no symptoms at all (89).

The source of the infection is often unknown. In some cases bacteria in the blood proved to be the cause; other causes include skin ulcers resulting from vasculitis and infected rheumatoid nodules.

Important risk factors are a protracted and aggressive disease process (in most cases the RA will have lasted for more than 10 years (91)), extra-articular symptoms such as nodules and generalized vasculitis and Felty's syndrome (shortage of white blood cells). It is one of the most important complications in joint-replacement operations.

If treated at an early stage the septic arthritis usually takes a favourable course, although generally serious damage to the affected joints occurs later (67, 71). If the therapy is not instituted swiftly enough the prognosis is often poor (92), leading to total destruction of the joint and even death.

In five different surveys the percentage of (living or deceased) RA-patients who had at sometime or other suffered from septic arthritis varied from 0.3% to 3%. The incidence in a hospital population in one survey amounted to 0.5% of the RA-patients per year (91). The increasing use of steroids and immunosuppressives may be related to the rising incidence of infections (93).

Numerically, bacterial infections (e.g. septic arthritis and also urinary tract infections and pneumonia) are the most important cause of excess mortality among RA-patients (58). In a Canadian study in 1986, 13% of all mortality among RA-patients was attributed to sepsis or infections, compared with just 6% amount the population in general (31). Late diagnosis of the complication is a significant factor in this respect.

A number of foreign researchers have examined the prognosis for RA-patients with infected joints (i.e. spectic arthritis). If the various surveys are aggregated, the figures suggest that 45% of the patients recover completely, 19% die as a result of this complication and 36% continue to suffer from seriously affected joints (91). In a Dutch survey conducted among 44 RA-patients with septic arthritis, a complete recovery occurred among only 10%, 20% died while 70% continue to suffer impairment (94).

2.2.2.4 Iatrogenic Complications

By iatrogenic complications are meant the occurrence of complications resulting from medical and/or surgical treatment.

The drugs used in the treatment of RA may be divided into "non-steroid anti-inflammatory drugs" (NSAIDs) and "disease modifying anti-rheumatic drugs" DMARDs) (See Appendix 1). Generally speaking the treatment is started with NSAIDs. These drugs help control the pain and stiffness and, to some extent, the inflammation but do not have any real impact on the course of the disease itself. For this reason it is often necessary to add a DMARD to the medication after some time: anti-malaria drugs, sulphasalazine, gold compounds or penicillamine. If these drugs are not sufficiently effective or have excessive side-effects, immunosuppressives (cytostatics) or cortico-steroids may be administered. The inflammation may be halted locally in one or more joints by injection with corticosteroids.

The use of drugs entails risks. The vast majority of medicines used frequently by an RA-patient can have many side-effects. In comparison with the therapeutic effectiveness, the risk of side-effects is generally high in RA (89). The disease modifying anti-rheumatic drugs, in particular, tend to be toxic. In a prospective study conducted among 186 RA-patients who began a medicinal therapy with DMARDs at an early stage, 17% were required to halt the therapy on account of side-effects. These patients switched to different DMARDs or continued with NSAIDs only (95).
The various side-effects for each group of drugs and therapy group are described below.

NSAIDs, including acetylsalicylates
The most common side-effects of NSAIDs are inflammation of the stomach lining and gastric ulcers, sometimes resulting in haemorrhaging. These side-

effects are often associated with nausea, vomiting and pain (89). Some 25-35% of users report (generally mild) gastric problems. Serious disorders arise among 0.2% of users (96).

Over 10% of NSAID-users suffer from side-effects on the central nervous system, such as noises in the ear (65), headaches, dizziness and psychological disturbance (e.g. depression). The incidence of renal impairments is low (89, 96). In some cases there is a reduced production of blood cells (58). Asthma attacks among RA-patients also suffering from CNSLD can be aggravated. An extended bleeding time can be a complicating factor in operations (89).

When such side-effects occur, a switch is generally made to another NSAID, in the hope that this will produce fewer problems. The "newer" NSAIDs are generally tolerated reasonably well (97).

DMARDs

Anti-malaria drugs
Although anti-malaria drugs are known to have an enormous number of side-effects, these are infrequent and tend to be mild (89). At current dosages only 5% of patients are required to suspend the treatment on account of side-effects (98). The most serious complication is a disorder of the retina, but this side-effect occurs only rarely at the present dosages. The deposition in the cornea of a metabolic product in the drug disappears after the treatment is suspended (89).

Sulphasalazine
Side-effects include headaches, changes in mood, nausea, epigastric tenderness, loss of appetite and general malaise. These complaints are often dose-dependent. Anaemia can also occur. Less frequent side-effects are a reduction in the white-cell count, serious skin disorders and inflammation of the liver. Infertility can occur among males. Recovery is possible for most of the side-effects (98).

Gold compounds
The most important side effect of gold therapy is reversible renal damage with loss of protein in the urine. The side-effect that causes most concern amount patients is rashes (89). In some cases the blood count will drop or there will be inflammation of the mucus membrane of the mouth (58).

After injection 30-40% of patients suffer from side-effects, in 10% of cases serious side-effects (98). In some 25% of cases treatment with gold therapy has to be suspended on account of the side-effects (58), for which reason frequent monitoring of blood counts and urine is required.

Penicillamine
As in the case of gold therapy, renal damage is the most important complication arising from the use of penicillamine (89). It occurs among 10-30% of the patients being treated with penicillamine, although recovery is generally possible (98). The blood count may also drop.

A specific feature of penicillamine is that it can result in a loss of taste. Other disorders may also arise, such as myasthenia gravis (muscle fatigue giving way to paralysis) (58).

Immunosuppressives
The administration of these drugs may result in a reduced production of blood cells. Other possible side-effects include baldness, inflammation of the bladder, infertility and shingles (71). The immunosuppressive cyclophosphamide can cause malignancies in the long term (89, 98). There are far fewer such indications for other immunosuppressives, but this possibility does need to be taken into account. Some immunosuppressives, including methotrexate, can result in damage to the liver (58, 89), although this seldom forms a clinical problem (99).

Use of the experimental cyclosporin results in serious renal impairment, which does not recover fully after cessation of therapy (100).

Corticosteroids
The oral or intramuscular use of corticosteroids can result in many different side-effects, for which reason great caution is in order in respect of protracted treatment (67, 89). The toxicity falls sharply, however, when they are administered in low doses (101). Comparatively frequent complications include osteoporosis, Cushing's syndrome and the thinning of the skin. The death of bone tissue in the hip (aseptic bone necrosis) is common in therapy with high doses of steroids (89). A well known side-effect is the reactivation of tuberculosis (58).

Corticosteroids may also be administered by means of intra-articular injections. These locally acting corticosteroids can result in soft tissue atrophy

(89). If injections are administered carelessly this can result in blood poisoning (sepsis).

Chemical/radiation synovectomy
Apart from surgery, inflamed synovial tissue can be killed off by means of intra-articular administration of chemical substances or radioactive nuclides. This technique entails a risk of leakage of the chemical substance or nuclide from the joint. In particular leakage of the nuclide can expose the regional lymphatic glands and the liver to short but intensive radiation (58).

Surgical therapy
The most important surgical therapy is joint replacement. Following a joint-replacement operation, RA-patients run an increased risk of infections of the joint prosthesis. If an infection does in fact arise this can have serious consequences (89). Infections cannot always be prevented but, if recognized at an early stage, can be treated while preserving the prosthesis. In the event of protracted infections the prosthesis will have to be removed, although a new one can be added at a later stage (102).

If the prosthesis fails to fit properly into the bone a new operation will often be needed. The often limited mobility and bearing capacity mean that an artificial joint in an RA-patient tends to last longer than a prosthesis in a non-RA-patient.

Although wear of the individual parts of a prosthesis have so far received little attention, this is certainly an important factor in knee and hip replacements. The consequences may include synovitis, an increased risk of infection and detachment of the prosthesis element (102).

2.2.2.5 Conclusion

Among all patients suffering from the disease, RA leads to disorders of the joints. Many regard pain, and the dependence that pain brings on others, as one of the major problems of the disease. If movement is impaired and deformities arise the patient's functional capacity will be further reduced.

The extra-articular manifestations which, at first sight, might appear less serious (such as chronic fatigue and respiratory infections) can nevertheless be a major factor as they are comparatively frequent and reduce the quality of life of RA-patients. The more serious extra-articular manifestations are less common, but the consequences for the patient can be very great, sometimes even resulting in death.

The medical treatment of RA is often burdensome, since fairly toxic medicines have to be administered at an early stage in the disease process. These often have side-effects. Surgical therapy, which commonly involves joint-replacement operations, is also a radical measure for the patient. High demands are therefore made on the standard of medical care.

2.2.3 Quality of life of RA-patients

2.2.3.1 Introduction

Apart from the prolongation of life, improving the quality of life has always been one of the major objectives of medical treatment. Few researchers, however, provide a precise definition of quality of life. In many cases it is equated with the concept of health or *general well-being*, as defined by the WHO (103, 104). This definition distinguishes three components: physical, psychological and social.

The scientific literature devotes a good deal of attention to the impact of RA on the quality of life. By measuring the components of the quality of life, an indication can be obtained concerning the consequences of the disease and the treatment for the patient. The patient's well-being can be determined by evaluation by patient themselves, someone close to the patient (e.g. spouse/-partner or a relative) or a carer. Since the focus is often on more subjective experiences such as pain, tiredness and fear, and because the significance of these experiences for the patient's daily life can vary considerably from person to person, it is desirable to ask patients themselves about their well-being (105).

There are various methods for determining the general well-being of patients. A simple one is simply to ask the patient how he himself perceives his quality of life at that point. The responses to this question correlate well with those obtained by more complex methods (106). This approach, however, suffers from the drawback that it is difficult to interpret the response since information on the various aspects of quality of life is lacking.

A commonly used method is to measure several components of quality of life simultaneously with the aid of a questionnaire. Over the course of time a very large number of questionnaires have been developed, for both written and oral questioning. Some concentrate especially on physical functioning, while others measure the entire range of quality-of-life aspects. Some questionnaires may be applied to various kinds of chronic disorders, while others have been specially developed for rheumatic diseases, especially RA (104).

A comparison on the various studies into the quality of life is complicated by the fact that various definitions and concepts of quality of life are used. In addition a wide range of differing measurement instruments are employed and differently constructed control groups - or no control groups whatever - are used. Furthermore many instruments are incapable of measuring small changes in a person's functioning, although for the individual concerned such changes may have a major bearing. Many studies also suffer from the disadvantage that the research group is small. Most are, moreover, cross-sectional studies; only a few are longitudinal, and even then the follow-up period tends to be comparatively short.

Quality of life, and the components of quality of life, may be affected by a number of factors. The latter may be divided into influencing and intermediate (intervening) factors. These factors are shown schematically in highly simplified form in Chart 2.3.

From the chart it may be seen that the quality of life of an RA-patient is influenced by three groups of intervening factors, namely the somatic features of the disorder, the patient's coping capacity and the obtained social support. These three factors are in turn affected by other variables, such as personality characteristics, the quality of the RA care, patient education, societal developments, public information and the attitude of society towards sickness in general and RA in particular. The various elements of Chart 2.3 are examined briefly below (going from right to left).

Although the physical, psychological and social well-being will be examined in three separate sections below, this classification is an artificial one since the various components are mutually interactive. Furthermore, in the case of certain consequences of the disorder it is not always possible clearly to indicate to which of the three components they relate. An example is the recently described phenomenon that RA-patients devote a substantial proportion of their lives to matters related to their illness, such as extra rest and sleep, physiotherapy and visits to the doctor. In rough terms it has been calculated that RA-patients have on average 1870 fewer hours a year (32%) in terms of effective living than a healthy person (107). This loss of time can have an effect on both psychological and social well being.

Schedule 2.3 **Influencing and intervening factors and components of quality of life (well-being) of RA-patients**

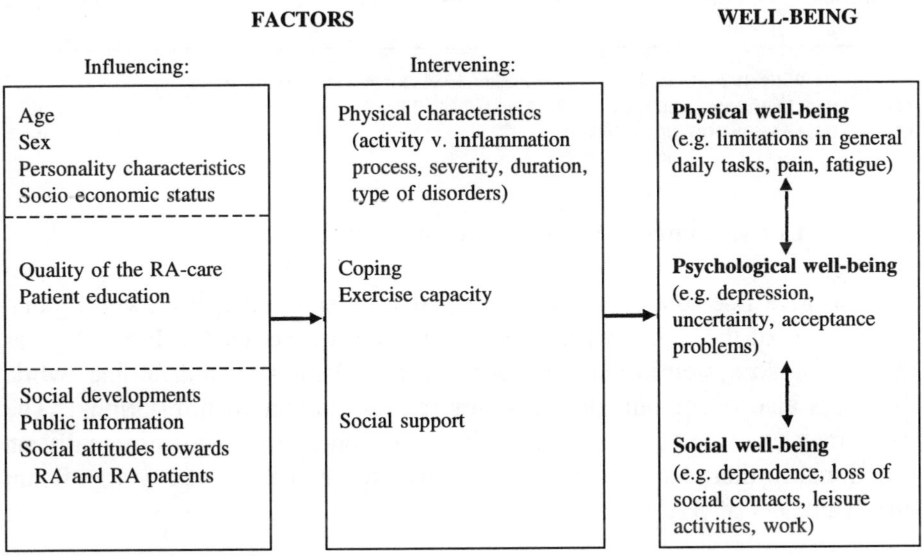

The results of four Dutch studies, each of which is concerned with quality of life, are discussed below in the following three sections. Various features of these studies are set out in Table 2.7. A more detailed account of these surveys and their limitations may be found in section 2.2.4.1. Findings from foreign studies in the field of the three dimensions of quality of life are discussed in section 2.4.3.

Table 2.7 Dutch studies in which quality-of-life aspects of (among others) RA-patients are examined

Study*	Research group	Number of patients	Percentage of women	Average age in years	Average duration of illness	Functional capacity (%) I	II	III	IV
De Witte	Rheum. Assoc.	179	79	61	15	-	-	-	-
Cornelissen	Outpatients	202	70	62	15	1	35	52	12
Rasker	Outpatients	203	52	55-65	8	9	65	15	0***
Meyboom-de Jong	General practice	23	61	68	5-15	0	48	30	22

* De Witte 1989, Cornelissen 1984, Rasker 1984, Meyboom-de-Jong 1989.
** For significance: see section 2.2.3.2 and Table 2.8.
*** Unknown in 10% of cases.

2.2.3.2 Consequences of RA for physical well-being

RA can give rise to articular disorders such as pain, stiffness, swelling and deformities of the joints, with a consequent loss of movement. In most cases there are also systemic features such as general malaise and fatigue, while disorders also occur outside the joints (extra-articular manifestations). The latter may even be to the forefront. This section concentrates especially on functional limitations. Pain and fatigue, which are cited as highly significant disadvantages of RA, were discussed in section 2.2.2.

In order to indicate the effect of these articular features and extra-articular manifestations of RA for physical functioning in a more readily understood manner, an instrument was developed as early as 1937, known as the Steinbröcker scale (108), which seeks to classify patients on the basis of their case histories and physical examination. The scale runs from 1 to 4 and provides a measure of the functional capacity or the ability to function in daily life (see Table 2.8). Although this classification is very broad it continues to be applied on account of its useability.

The survey conducted among members of the Netherlands Rheumatism Association revealed that 43% of the RA-patients regarded the disorder as serious or very serious, 41% regarded it as moderately serious and 16% as slight or not serious. As far as the activities of daily living were concerned the main problems experienced by RA-patients proved to be in the field of household tasks and activities in and outside the house, walking, recreation and leisure. A comparatively high proportion of RA-patients (in comparison with other rheumatic disorders) had difficulty in coping with specific activities such as walking at the same pace as before (69%), performing heavy activities in and about the house (68%), standing for any length of time (58%), writing or typing (49%), using public transport (48%) and participating in group activities (35%). In addition many RA-patients turned out to need help for activities in which they had to use their hands. One striking finding was that half the patients no longer rode a bicycle and a quarter had difficulty in doing so (109).

Table 2.8 Functional capacity in classes according to the classification of the American Rheumatism Association

Class	Functional capacity	Criteria
I	Undisturbed	Complete functional capacity with ability to carry on all usual duties without handicaps
II	Adequate	Functional capacity adequate to conduct normal activities despite discomfort or limited mobility of one or more joints
III	Limited	Functional capacity adequate to perform only a limited number of the duties of usual occupation or self-care
IV	Complete dependence	Total or almost total incapacitation, with patients bedridden or confined to wheelchair, able to perform little or no self-care.

Source: 58, based on 108

The survey conducted by Cornelissen among 202 patients suffering either from RA with walking problems (84%) or osteoarthrosis with walking problems (16%) revealed that the patients were less mobile than individuals in the matched control group drawn from the population registers in a number of municipalities. Fewer patients cycled, the distance that they were able to walk without resting was shorter and they visited public buildings and shops less frequently. The mobility of urban-dwellers was consistently lower than that of village-dwellers (110).

Most of the RA-patients in Rasker's survey were able to carry out the general activities of daily life wholly independently. Help was needed especially in dressing and undressing, showering and taking a bath and going up and down stairs. In respect of each of these activities 35% of the RA-patients nevertheless needed some form of special appliances or help from other persons to a greater of lesser extent. The remainder were able to carry out these activities independently.

Nearly 20% of the patients considered *themselves* that they suffered from a serious form of arthritis, a little over 25% referred to it as "a comparatively serious form", while 52% regarded it as "not so serious".

The majority of the patients (69%) had major problems when it came to heavy household work. Three-quarters were able to cope reasonably well with lighter household work, although 64% of these patients did at times find it more difficult to cope. The inability to carry out daily work or hobbies, or to do so only with discomfort and difficulty, was cited by a quarter of the patients as the biggest drawback of the disease (64).

As in the case of the survey conducted among members of the Rheumatism Association, the survey conducted by Meyboom-de Jong also revealed that the major problem in terms of daily physical functioning centered on housework and activities in and about the house, recreation, leisure and walking. Sleeping and resting, mobility and travel and bodily care and movement were also less than optimal. In specifying their own physical condition 9% said that they were still capable of substantial exertion, 26% that they were slightly or moderately limited and 65% that they were capable of little if any physical exertion. With respect to the activities of daily living 4% considered themselves unimpeded, 78% were somewhat to moderately impeded and 17% considerably impeded. Nobody said that they were very seriously incapacitated by the RA. In respect of both aspects the group of RA-patients was significantly more limited than the total group of elderly persons (111, 112).

To sum up it may be concluded that:

1. A high proportion of the RA-patients have difficulty with activities requiring any degree of exertion or for which they need to use their hands. The figure varies from 35% to 70%, depending on the research group and activity.

2. Problems were encountered particularly with heavier household tasks, walking, standing for any length of time, going up and down stairs, shopping and travelling by public transport.
3. The majority of the patients sometimes have great difficulty in managing their daily activities.

2.2.3.3 Consequences of RA for psychological well-being

Among other things the psychological consequences of RA for the patient depend on age and the particular situation he or she faces. Each life-cycle stage involves its own characteristic questions, cares and problems. Nevertheless the way in which RA-patients experience their condition has much in common. In general the psychological consequences of RA manifest themselves particularly in feelings of depression, uncertainty about the future and problems concerning acceptance.

A Dutch survey revealed that both physical and psychological aspects (i.e. fear and depression) contributed independently of one another to the way in which RA-patients experience their health (113).

The survey conducted by the Netherlands Rheumatism Association showed that RA-patients experienced the most problems with bodily activities. These did not automatically affect psychological well-being (i.e. emotional behaviour and alertness/intellectual functioning), although 18% of the RA-patients did suffer from feelings of depression and 13% felt that there was little for him or her to be proud about. These percentages were somewhat higher than those for the other diagnostic groups (i.e. osteoarthrosis, ankylosing spondylitis and fibrositis). RA-patients were gloomier about their future prospects than others: 21% viewed the future optimistically, 50% were neutral and 29% pessimistic. In addition 45% expected that matters would be worse in two years' time (109).

The survey conducted by Cornelissen asked whether people were satisfied with the present situation. Of the patients 53% said that they were, compared with 88% of the controls (110).

In the survey conducted by Rasker, patients were asked whether they accepted the disease as something they had to live with. Of the patients 72% said that they accepted the disease. Elderly people appeared more reconciled to their situation than young people. Approximately a quarter of the RA-patients said that they still had difficulty in accepting the disease. Many of those who said that they had now come to terms with the disease indicated that they had had considerable difficulty in doing so in the past. Problems included lack of familiarity with the disease, trying to understand how it had been contracted, fitting the disease into the patient's life and the uncertain future. Fear of discomfort and an increased severity of the disease were also factors. Of the patients 90% considered life to be worthwhile and nearly three-quarters were in fact very happy. A third often entertained worries about the future, while half did not (64).

The Meyboom-de Jong survey also revealed that most of the problems encountered by RA-patients related to physical activities and much less so to psychological activities (i.e. emotional behaviour and alertness/intellectual functioning). In indicating their own psychological condition, 26% said that they were unaware of any limitations, 65% felt that they were somewhat or moderately limited and 9% said that they were limited (111).

To sum up it may be concluded that:

1. If RA-patients experience limitations in their functional capacity this does not necessarily mean that there are also psychological problems.
2. RA-patients suffer somewhat more frequently from feelings of depression than patients with a different rheumatic disorder.
3. A comparatively high proportion of the patients are concerned about the future.
4. RA-patients are less satisfied than non-RA-patients.
5. Many patients have had difficulty in accepting the disease.

2.2.3.4 Consequences of RA for social well-being

Limitations in mobility may result in dependence and loss of *social contacts* and hence in isolation. The ability to obtain practical and/or emotional support depends on the quantity and quality of social contacts. Because RA-patients often need such support, the social network plays a significant role.

In the survey conducted among members of the Netherlands Rheumatism Association, it appeared that the extent of problems encountered with physical activities did not have any direct consequences for social functioning (i.e. social interaction and communication). Nevertheless 35% of the RA-patients participated less frequently in group-based activities than they did hitherto. Only 3% experienced problems in their relationships with their partners, which was less than the figure for other diagnostic groups with which the RA-patients were compared.

RA-patients turned out not to be notably lonely in comparison with the Dutch population in general (113). The most practical and emotional support was received from the partner and then from the children, and the least support from other relatives. A notably high level of emotional support was obtained from fellow-sufferers, although this may well reflect the composition of the research group, consisting as it did of members of rheumatic patient associations (109).

The Cornelissen survey did not detect any difference in the frequency of interaction with relatives and friends between patients and controls. Despite the roughly equal frequency of the interaction, 35% of the patients had the feeling that the number of social contacts had fallen since the onset of the disorder, while 5% felt they had increased. Patients in urbanized areas had a greater need for social interaction than patients from rural areas.

Patients received a greater level of informal help from other members of the household than did controls. Among the patient group some 60% indicated that they received a considerable amount of help from other members of the household. Other important sources of informal help were friends and acquaintances. One noteworthy finding was that neighbours proved to play a subordinate role in the provision of informal help.

In addition 50% of the patients felt they were dependent on the help of other family members and 55% felt awkward about asking for such help from those around them. One of the major drawbacks experienced as a result of the disease was, consequently, dependence: for 25% this was the largest single drawback. Dependence may also be related to the inability to cope with all the activities people were formerly able to perform. For 41% this was the biggest problem (110).

The Rasker survey asked a number of questions about social interaction. Of the RA-patients 29% said that they seldom or never went to visit other people. In 40% of these cases the reason cited was RA. Some 10% often felt lonely and depressed. Among 21% of the patients the disease had affected their relationship with their partner, with much the same numbers reporting a deterioration as an improvement. Problems were experienced in sexual contact and the partner often displayed lack of understanding about the effects of the disease. Among 19% of the patients with a family the disease had caused problems in the family. Dependence was regarded as one of the major drawbacks of the disease by 37% of the RA-patients (64).

The Meyboom-de Jong survey similarly showed that RA-patients encountered most problems with respect to functional capacity and far fewer in relation to social functioning. In specifying their own social condition (i.e. the extent to which they were able to maintain contacts with family, acquaintances and clubs) 43% said that they were unrestricted, 39% somewhat or moderately restricted and 17% restricted (111).

As emerged previously from the Rasker survey, a proportion of the RA-patients encounter problems in their *sexual contacts*. Sexual activity is hampered by discomfort, numbness, fatigue and restricted mobility. Psychological changes, such as depression and a loss of self-esteem, can also reduce the libido and energy. Complications of the disorder can result to specific problems in the sexual sphere. Sjögren's syndrome, for example, is associated with a dry vagina. A number of studies revealed a decline in sexual activity among the majority of patients since the onset of RA. A survey conducted among women, for example, indicated that over half had suffered a loss of libido and that the frequency of sexual intercourse had fallen. Some patients also had problems in achieving orgasm (114). Another Dutch study revealed that there was more aversion to sexual activity among RA-patients than among healthy individuals or patients suffering from ankylosing spondylitis. The aversion was more marked among patients in an active stage of the disease. Foreplay was significantly briefer and RA-patients enjoyed sexual activity less frequently (115).

The disorder means that RA-patients often have to give up or reduce their work. In some cases they have difficulty finding adapted work. As a result of sickness absence and employment disability they lose social contacts and also suffer financially.

The Central Bureau of Statistics (116) provides information on the extent of *sickness absence* from paid employment. In 1987 a diagnostic code was assigned by a medical insurance officer in 28% of sickness absence cases. Of these 0.11% related to RA. A strikingly high number of cases - 2.3% - were recorded under the heading "other or not further examined joint involvements". It may be that a proportion of the sickness absence due to RA could not be diagnosed as such by the medical insurance officer. It is therefore reasonable to assume that a proportion of the sickness absence recorded in this residual category consists of absence as a result of RA. If in calculating the absolute number of sickness absence cases an adjustment is made for the rate of participation in the CBS statistics and absences that did not result in the payment of benefits (under the waiting-period regulations), RA then turns out to have accounted for some 10,150 cases of absence in 1987. The category of "other or not further investigated joint involvements" accounted for some 214,000 cases of absence in 1987.

The survey conducted among members of the Netherlands Rheumatism Association also asked about *employment disability*. Of the 107 RA-patients aged under 65, 90% said they were not working. Of these 51% said they were not working as a result of RA. In this survey 66% of the 207 rheumatism patients (lumping all the diagnostic categories together) aged under 65 said that they had been officially classed as disabled, most of them (81%) with an invalidity rate of over 80%. Of those officially classed as suffering from employment disability, 70% said that they were fully and 23% partially classed as disabled as a result of the rheumatic disorder. A substantial proportion (28%) of the patients not working as a result of rheumatism (again lumping all diagnostic categories together) indicated that they were perfectly capable of working partially or with adaptations. In addition 40% said that they were anxious or very anxious to work, while 21% did not care either way (109).

Although the survey conducted by Rasker asked few detailed questions concerning work-related aspects, it nevertheless revealed that 30% of the men with RA and 28% of the women with RA had ceased paid employment on account of the illness (it was not specified whether that illness was RA), while 22% and 15% respectively were still in employment. Of the latter groups, 16% and 41% respectively had a certain amount of difficulty in working - men more than women (64).

Employment disability data issued by the Joint Medical Service (117) indicate that in 1988 RA was the cause (i.e. principal diagnosis) of roughly 0.8% of the total number of persons drawing invalidity benefit. These do not include figures from the General Civil Servants' Superannuation Fund. In absolute terms the figure of 0.8% covered nearly 6,100 persons (aged 15-65). Nearly half were aged 55-65. Annually some 480 individuals are declared unfit as a result of RA. This applies especially in middle age: approximately 70% of those declared unfit are aged between 40 and 59. The total number of new invalidity benefit claimants as a result of RA in terms of both main and subsidiary diagnosis in 1988 was around 520. Roughly the same number of men as women were declared unfit as a result of RA.

In the Rheumatism Association and Rasker surveys the patients were asked to estimate the additional costs. Foreign surveys have revealed that these estimates correspond closely with the actual additional costs (118).

In the Rheumatism Association survey, respondents were asked whether they were financially less well off as a result of the disorder. Two-thirds said that they were, while one third said that it made no difference. No distinction was drawn in terms of diagnostic groups. In addition 87% of the rheumatism patients turned out to have additional costs, the most common items being medicines, physiotherapy, household/nursing help and additional electricity/-heating charges. The most expensive items for the respondent (after the deduction of reimbursements) were household/nursing help and special aids and facilities inside and outside the house. Less but still expensive were additional electricity/heating costs, clothing, visits to health farms, special dietary requirements, travel costs and physiotherapy. Here again no classification was made in terms of diagnostic groups. The total average annual additional costs per RA-patient were NLG 1,758 (109).

Respondents also emphasized their difficult financial circumstances in the Rasker survey. No reimbursements are provided for the costs of certain facilities, medicines or alternative forms of treatment that appeared beneficial, and the patients themselves could not afford them. Nearly a third felt that they were worse off financially as a result of the illness. A little over half, however, did not take that view. The average additional costs as a result of having RA amounted to NLG 1,462 a year. These costs were not reimbursed out of insurance or subsidies. The most common costs were travel expenses, medicines, clothing and footwear. The most expensive items for the patients were travel expenses, household/nursing help, clothing/footwear, special aids and appliances and special dietary requirements (64).

To sum up it may be concluded that:

1. RA-patients whose functional capacity is impaired do not always encounter problems in their social functioning.
2. RA-patients are not notably lonely. The frequency of social contacts is roughly the same or slightly smaller than that of controls.
3. Dependence is regarded as a major drawback.

4. The most practical and emotional support is received from the partner and children.
5. The major problems are nevertheless encountered in the relationship with the patient's partner (i.e. lack of understanding concerning the consequences of the disease), in sexual activity and family life.
6. A high proportion of the RA-patients do not work or have been declared unfit for work as a result of RA. Those in employment sometimes have difficulty performing their work.
7. A substantial proportion of those no longer working would be perfectly able to work partially or if adaptations were made.
8. In 1987 there were at least 10,150 cases of sickness absence as a result of RA.
9. Nearly 6,100 persons were declared unfit for work in 1988 on account of RA. Some 520 individuals are declared unfit for work each year as a result of RA.
10. RA-patients incur substantial additional costs as a result of their illness, averaging around NLG 1,500 a year.

2.2.3.5 Factors affecting the quality of life

This section briefly examines the influencing and intervening factors. A number of foreign studies have investigated the way in and extent to which influencing and intervening factors are related to the quality of life. The results of some of these studies are also discussed below.

Intervening factors

Chart 2.3 shows three factors that affect the quality of life, namely the physical characteristics of the disorder, the patient's coping capacity and the obtained social support.

The *physical characteristics* cover the activity of the inflammation process, the severity and duration of the disease, articular features, extra-articular manifestations and handicaps.

Most patients and carers assume that psychosocial factors are related to aspects of the disease such as functional limitations and discomfort. On account of measurement problems and methodological shortcomings, studies into this suggested relationship have so far failed to produce clearcut results (119).

Similarly the duration and severity of the disorder turn out to be related in some surveys to functional limitations and/or psychological well-being and not in others. American studies revealed that the demonstrable somatic severity of the disease is not closely correlated with the extent of subjectively experienced complaints, psychological well-being or functional capacity (120, 121). Nor was any link established between the duration of the disease and psychological well-being (122), although the duration and functional limitations were related (123). By contrast other recent studies into the impact of chronic diseases indicate that the duration of the disorders significantly affects the psychological and social well-being.

In this respect three periods are broadly distinguished. Kraaimaat has formulated this classification more specifically for RA-patients (124). In the first two years of the disease the main emphasis of the patient lies on obtaining information on his illness and coming to terms with it. During the first three to 20 years of the disorder the emphasis is on adapting to a generally gradual deterioration. Once the disease has lasted more than 20 years ageing processes become a significant factor, manifesting themselves in an acceleration and deterioration of the physical, psychological and social condition.

In a large longitudinal study in Canada among 681 RA-patients who were followed for a period of at least eight years, it was shown that limitations in the activities of daily life developed most rapidly in the early years of the disease. Later the progression is much slower (125). Similarly Meenan found that the health condition (i.e. discomfort and physical and psychological condition) of a group of patients who had had RA for some years remained fairly stable over a five-year period (126). Other surveys, by contrast, indicate a loss in functional capacity over a lengthier period (17, 127).

A Dutch cross-sectional survey indicated that the majority of the clinical and laboratory findings were related to the physical aspects of health perception. They are not however related to the psychological and social aspects (128). In both cross-sectional and longitudinal foreign studies it was found that psychological factors are, to a greater extent than factors providing a measure of the disease activity, related to the extent in which people are able to perform the activities of daily life (123, 129, 130).

The patient's *coping capacity* also affects the quality of life. Relevant factors in this respect include the extent of acceptance of the disorder (going through the "mourning process") and satisfaction with the residual functional capacity, dealing with stress (e.g. an uncertain future, relationship problems, employment) and the ways found of living with the disease.

A survey conducted among 361 RA-patients found that an active response to pain (e.g. distracting attention from the discomfort) is associated with a lower level of depression, pain and physical impairment. Passive ways of dealing with pain (e.g. reducing social activities) were associated with more depression, pain and physical limitation (131). A number of other studies also found that a "negative" response to the disease, manifesting itself for example in unrealistic expectations (fantasies) or blaming oneself instead of fitting the disease into daily life, was associated with a poor psychological state and greater functional impairment (119, 132). Patients who are unable to reflect realistically on their situation and who are unable to adjust their goals evidently encounter more frequent psychological problems as a result of their RA.

A British study carried out in 1988 revealed that psychological well-being was in large measure determined by the RA-patient's satisfaction with his functional capabilities. That satisfaction was in turn dependent on the comparison drawn by the patient between his own ability to function and that of both healthy persons and other RA-patients (133). The process of acceptance of and adaptation to the disease also determined the extent to which people were limited (123). Feelings of depression were found to be associated with the degree of pain, blood sedimentation rate, stiffness and satisfaction with other aspects of life (134).

A Dutch survey conducted by Kraaimaat revealed that pain was closely associated with physical functioning. The degree of stress (fear, gloominess) was not related to the degree of pain. The fact that little if any correlation was found between pain and stress means that the two aspects require separate attention in the treatment of RA-patients. In addition certain coping strategies proved to have a favourable effect on the perceived pain and stress but an unfavourable effect on physical functioning. It was concluded that the short and long-term effects of coping can be in opposition (135).

The fact that dependence is such an significant component of social well-being shows the importance of *social support*. The extent of social support is determined by whether or not the individual concerned forms part of a social network, the existence of supporting interactions (i.e. the number of interactions and discrepancy between obtained and desired interactions) and the feeling of obtaining support (or perceived support) (136). Studies reveal the patient's partner to be the most important source of support in chronic diseases. The partner provides both practical and emotional support. Help from children or other relatives cannot be so readily assumed. While such help will be forthcoming in one-off and emergency situations, such as admission to hospital, the provision of help by children becomes problematic once there is a permanent need for help in daily activities (137). These findings also apply in the case of RA-patients (see section 2.2.3.4 on social well-being). In general it is assumed that social support contributes towards good physical or psychological well-being. Some research data, however, also suggest a negative correlation; in these cases the social support actually undermines the patient's health by interfering with or detracting from personal autonomy, thus placing the person who is receiving support even more in the role of patient (137). Social support is also discussed in section 5.2.4.1 concerning informal care.

Influencing factors

The three intervening factors described above are in turn determined by a large number of other factors. A number of these factors provide scope for intervention to improve the quality of life. Examples include the quality of the treatment of the RA-patient, patient information and education, activities to promote self-reliance, socio-political developments, public education and the associated attitude of society towards RA and RA-patients. In addition there are factors where little if any intervention is possible, such as age, sex, certain personal characteristics and socio-economic status.

Possibilities for improving the medical care provided to RA-patients, including patient education, are discussed in section 4.5 concerning the policy scenario. Economic austerity, as an example of a socio-political development, is further elaborated in one of the alternative scenarios (section 4.4).

The fact that various surveys have found that psychosocial factors exert a marked effect on the course taken by the disease and the extent of impairment in daily activities provides a case for paying greater attention to those factors. In this respect *patient information and education* play a significant role, especially education; information by itself will rarely lead to an improvement in health (138).

It is important for patients to learn how to control their daily lives themselves. One problem in this regard is that RA often takes a variable, unpredictable course, so that patients tend to regard their illness as uncontrollable (139). The result can be that patients downgrade the effectiveness of self-care and develop feelings of helplessness (140). Research has shown that patient education that helps patients acquire self-care skills can help them deal more effectively with the consequences of the disorder, ultimately leading to improved well-being (141). In this regard social support can help increase the patient's self-care capacity (142). Especially in the United States successful education programmes have been developed for patients with rheumatic disorders (143), but similar programmes for RA-patients also now exist in the Netherlands (144, 145). So far these have been group programmes but an individual programme is also being developed aimed at strengthening self-care. Protocols are also being developed for carers aimed at the improved coordination of and continuity in patient education and information (146).

A significant influencing factor for the quality of life consists of the *social attitudes* towards RA. Until recently, and since at least 1942, researchers have been trying to identify an "RA-specific personality", on the assumption that a large number of negative personality traits could be a significant factor in the onset of RA (120, 138). Fortunately this idea no longer holds sway. Although no research data are available on the subject, it is possible that negative notions about RA-patients of this kind still persist in Dutch society. What is clear is that a number of problems faced by RA-patients are generally not acknowledged by those around them. It is, for example, not generally known that pain and dependence can have major consequences for psychological or social functioning. Another problem is that patients are sometimes not taken seriously but are regarded with suspicion because the severity of the complaints can vary from day to day or even from moment to moment (64). Finally, a number of prejudices towards rheumatism (including RA) are a factor. Rheumatism is for example often regarded as a disease of old age about which nothing can be done (147).

Efforts to improve public attitudes towards RA and RA-patients can be made by means of public education.

2.2.3.6 Conclusion

On the basis of the information outlined above RA may be said to detract from the quality of life. This applies to both the physical, psychological and the social component. The extent of the negative impact depends, however, on a large number of factors, such as the somatic characteristics of the disorder, the patient's ability to accept the disease and fit it into daily life and the social support he or she receives.

The consequences of RA outlined in this section broadly correspond with the consequences that chronic disorders generally involve. Turk (148) has described how chronic illnesses are often associated with permanent changes in physical functioning, feelings of fear, depression and helplessness, isolation from family and friends, loss of significant roles and positions and the disruption of plans for the future.

There are various possibilities for improving the quality of life for RA-patients. These include a reduction in the somatic severity of the disorder (e.g. by adequate RA care), increasing the resilience of the patient (e.g. by patient education, remedial therapy and enhancing self-reliance), changing negative attitudes within society towards RA-patients (e.g. by public education) and official measures to improve the financial situation and conditions of employment. The care covers a very wide range of fields and it is important for it to be provided effectively, with an absence of gaps, contradictions and overlap. To this end effective cooperation between the various carers is vital so that the respective forms of care can be coordinated and integrated with one another. Apart from positive effects on the quality of life of the patient and the latter's family this may also have a beneficial effect on the course of the disease and the level of medical consumption.

2.2.4 Medical consumption as a result of RA

2.2.4.1 Introduction

By medical consumption is meant the extent to which patients with rheumatoid arthritis make use of health care facilities as a result of suffering from the disease. The term "as a result of" means that the use of health care facilities arises from having RA. All other forms of consumption by RA-patients, such as the general uptake of medical care, are not described in this section since this would provide an incorrect impression of the uptake of care attributable to rheumatoid arthritis. The choice of information sources has accordingly been limited to those surveys in which the reason for the medical consumption could be attributed to rheumatoid arthritis. Use has been made of data from the literature, information obtained from institutes where studies have not yet been completed or published and information from institutes that do not publish the specific data required.

The figures presented in this section constitute a **baseline** for the total uptake of care resulting from rheumatoid arthritis. The figures are a bottom limit because the sources of information consulted tend to underreport the level of consumption for the following reasons:

1. A proportion of the RA-patients are not diagnosed as such (cf. the difference in prevalence between the EPOZ survey and NUHI records). It is however possible that these patients make use of care facilities as a result of the (as yet undiscovered) disorder. The consumption of these unknown RA-patients is not, however, included when determining the uptake of care.
2. A certain level of consumption takes place that is not directly the result of rheumatoid arthritis but where the disease has been a significant causal or contributory factor. Examples include medical consumption of RA-patients as a result of respiratory infections, fractures (resulting from osteoporosis) or as a result of side-effects of anti-rheumatoid drugs, as well as consumption generated in a much more indirect manner (e.g. a higher level of care in families containing RA-patients on account of the heavier demands made on informal care).
3. In some cases the consumption arising directly from rheumatoid arthritis is incorrectly assigned in the records to a different diagnosis. This is due to differences in interpretation with respect to the diagnosis of rheumatoid arthritis (among both patients and carers).

Where a large measure of underreporting is suspected, the total consumption of RA-patients in comparison with that of non-RA-patients has been shown in certain places in this report (e.g. in relation to GP care).

One notable finding is the fact that there are no large-scale reliable surveys that describe the uptake of care by RA-patients. In order to provide an overall impression of the uptake of care it was necessary to draw on a number of sources. The latter do not, however, collect the data in a uniform manner. The studies differ in terms of survey methods, population size, representativeness and diagnostic criteria, etc.. It is vitally important to take these differences into account in interpreting the data presented in this section.

The results of seven sources of information are repeatedly drawn upon in this section. To avoid undue repetition, a brief description of the various studies is provided below.

1. Survey among members of the Netherlands Rheumatism Association (109):
   As part of the tenth anniversary celebrations of the Netherlands Federation of Associations of Patients with Rheumatic Disorders, a survey was conducted among 372 rheumatism patients (response rate: 74%) who were members of the Rheumatism Association (the number of RA-patients was 179). The results of this survey are not however representative since patients who were not a member of the Rheumatism Association are not represented in the research group. In addition it could be argued that the survey method (i.e. completing a detailed questionnaire) prevented patients with more serious or extensive rheumatic disorders from filling in the questionnaire and that they were consequently underrepresented.

2. Cornelissen survey (110):
   On the basis of a questionnaire Cornelissen conducted interviews with 170 RA and 32 arthrosis patients with walking problems who were living in or around the town of Enschede (response rate: 94%). All the patients were under treatment at the local rheumatology clinic. A distinction was drawn between urban and rural patients. The patients were compared with a control group (drawn from the population register) matched in terms of age and sex. The patient group is not representative of the total group of RA-patients since patients not being treated by the rheumatologist were not included in the research group. In addition a proportion of the patient group in question consisted of arthrosis sufferers, although no significant differences were detected between RA and arthrosis patients.

3. Rasker survey (64):
   In a survey conducted among a sample of 203 RA-patients (response rate: 86%) drawn from the address lists of two rheumatology centres in Amsterdam and Groningen, oral interviews were also conducted on the basis of a questionnaire. In this survey the patients were divided into a physically less and a physically more dependent group. Once again it should be noted that in view of the way in which the patients were selected they are not representative of RA-patients in general.

4. CBS Health Interview Survey (149):
   The CBS annually conducts oral interviews with a representative sample of the population (absolute response in 1989 approx. 8,500 persons). In 1989 the respondents were asked whether they suffered from "osteoarthritis (i.e. chronic rheumatism, RA) of the hands or feet". Apart from this category there were also separate categories for back complaints, wear and tear of the joints and a residual category of "other chronic rheumatic disorders lasting more than three months". Of the 8,500 respondents, 2.3% indicated in 1989 that they suffered from "osteoarthritis (i.e. chronic rheumatism, RA) of the hand or feet" (198 persons). In the remainder of this section these individuals have been classified as RA-patients, but the diagnosis cannot be certain.

5. Ommoord Monitoring Project (150):
   This concerned a morbidity monitoring project conducted by 12 general practitioners in and around Rotterdam in 1979-1981, with a total practice population of around 21,000. Registration took place on the basis of face-to-face (GP-patients) contact. The limitation of this survey is the fact that RA-patients were only registered if they had consulted the general practitioner in a face-to-face contact concerning the disorder. Patients with disorders who were not seen by the general practitioner escaped the database.

6. Transition project (151):
   This was another morbidity monitoring project conducted in nine general practices (25 general practitioners) in 1986-1988, covering a total of around 40,000 person-years. The method of registration was the same as that in the Ommoord project.

7. Self-Sufficiency Project (111):
   Once again this was a morbidity monitoring project, carried out in the north of the Netherlands in 12 general practices (covering 25 general practitioners), but confined to the population aged over 65. The total research population consisted of some 5,500 individuals. Otherwise the method was the same as that used in the Ommoord and Transition Projects.

Before examining the uptake of professional care as a result of RA, two significant non-professional forms of care will first be discussed, namely *self-care and informal care*. By these forms of care is understood: "the care provided on a non-professional basis in respect of a person's own health and that of those close to him". Self-care and informal care are to some extent complementary to professional health care.

Self-care:
As in the case of other chronic disorders it is considered important for patients with rheumatoid arthritis to take personal responsibility for the disease and to develop self-care activities. In the first place self-care consists of following up therapy and medication advice, such as performing exercises and taking medicines at the right time and in the right way. Over half the RA-patients in the survey conducted among members of the Rheumatism Association (109) indicated that they exercised by themselves. On average they exercise 3.4 hours a week, spread over 5.5 days.

Medical compliance is briefly examined in the section dealing with the use of drugs. Self-care may, however, also be concerned with the observance of a certain regimen, such as adapting daily activities to the limitations imposed by the disease. A significant precondition for self-care is an adequate level of patient education, guidance and support.

Where they are required, the provision of appliances can help the RA-patient to function more independently. In the survey conducted among members of the Rheumatism Association (109), 64% of the RA-patients turned out to have one or more appliances at their disposal (on average 1.4 appliances per person). Appliances to improve mobility (such as crutches or a wheelchair), for personal care and protection (such as modified toilets and taps and a shower-seat) and adaptations in the home (such as handles, modified chairs, bed and kitchen) are mentioned the most frequently. Nearly a quarter of the respondents with appliances at their disposal had had problems in obtaining them (such as long waiting periods and no or only partial reimbursement).

In a survey conducted among RA-patients treated at an outpatient rheumatology clinic (64), 41% indicated that they used one or more appliances or had had adaptations fitted in connection with the disorder and 31% required an appliance or modification. The use of or need for appliances was greater among women than men.

In their responses to a questionnaire, 29% of the 182 RA-patients being treated at an outpatient rheumatology clinic (152) indicated that adaptations had been made in the home or at work. Over 30% indicated that they wanted adaptations or appliances. In the survey conducted by Cornelissen (110) among RA and arthrosis patients, 30-40% turned out to have at least one adaptation fitted in the home. In the vast majority of cases the patients had paid for these adaptations themselves. Of the patients covered by the survey, 10-25% wanted further adaptations to the home. A significant conclusion to emerge from this survey was that patients were not generally well informed of the possibilities in this field and sources of financial support. The controls interviewed as part of the survey, for example, even proved to be better informed than the rheumatic patients concerning the appliances available from the home-nursing association.

Informal care:
Informal care is the care provided to the patient by their partner, children, relatives and friends or by voluntary organizations. The help provided within the home - especially by the partner - is an extremely important aspect of informal care. Apart from the care provided to patients with serious, incapacitating forms of RA, informal care also includes helping the patient to carry out his or her responsibilities within the family situation or taking over those tasks on his or her behalf, as well as help of a more social and psychological nature, such as helping the patient to accept the disorder, and displaying understanding. The provision of information and education to those concerned is also of major importance in informal care. See also section 2.2.3.5.

2.2.4.2 Medical consumption as a result of RA

There is no primary prevention or curative treatment for RA. The treatment of rheumatoid arthritis is directed towards (153):

1. Combating the disease itself and limiting the damage to joints as far as possible.
2. Alleviation of pain and stiffness.
3. Maintenance of optimal mobility.
4. Adaptation (of the patient to the disease, of the environment to the patient and of the patient to the environment).

Apart from measures directed towards the patient and the disorder, the treatment schedule therefore also contains measures to modify the home and work environment with a view to overcoming functional problems at home and in society.

The treatment of RA-patients consists of a number of elements (153, 154):

1. Dosed rest, especially in the active phases of the disease (e.g. bed-rest, immobilizing splints).
2. Physiotherapy and especially remedial therapy (e.g. active and passive movement and the application of heat/cold).
3. Psychological guidance and support.
4. Medicinal drugs.
5. Ergotherapy (i.e. measures to protect the joints).
6. Surgical treatment.

Patient education is a significant aspect of all these forms of treatment. Various carers are involved in the treatment.

Chart 2.4 indicates the various medical consumption possibilities for RA-patients. On account of the multi-facetted and protracted nature of the disorder, the RA-patient may come into contact with a large number of carers and institutions.

Although no breakdown into the various rheumatic disorders could be provided, the survey conducted among members of the Rheumatism Association (109) indicated that on average rheumatic patients came into contact with 2.9 different carers on an annual basis as a result of the disorder (primary health care: average of 1.7; secondary health care: average of 1.2). In the case of the annual number of contacts with professional carers a breakdown by diagnosis was possible. The median annual number of contacts of RA-patients with professional carers was 28, i.e. some two contacts per month.

The chart draws a distinction between the consumption of drugs (I), medical care (II) and care facilities (III). Within these categories a further distinction is drawn between primary, secondary and tertiary care. By primary care is meant non-hospital care, by secondary care outpatient treatment and non-ambulant (clinical) care. Tertiary care covers on the one hand care institutions of a specialized nature and on the other facilities preceded by primary or secondary care.

Although numerous sources of information were available, it was not possible to quantify the volume of consumption for each kind of facility. The lack of reliable information meant that the role of rest-homes in the care of RA-patients could not be assessed.

Chart 2.4 Medical consumption possibilities for RA-patients

I *Drugs*

II *Medical assistance* (consultations, contacts)

Primary care	Secondary care
- general practitioner	- specialists (rheumatologist, internist, orthopaedist, pediatrician, plastic surgeon, neurologist, neurosurgeon, opthamalogist, dermatologist, rehabilitation doctor)
- physiotherapist	- ergotherapist
- district nurse/health visitor/ district rheumatology nurse	
- home help	
- social worker	
- alternative medicine practitioner	

III *Health care facilities* (hospital admissions, nursing/treatment days)

Secondary care	Tertiary care
- outpatient clinic (rheumatology, internal, pain clinic)	- (rheumatology) rehabilitation centre
- hospital	- nursing home
	- rest-home

In all probability the patterns of consumption vary considerably according to the severity of the rheumatoid arthritis. Unfortunately no data on consumption are available that link up with the various levels of severity.

The sources of information may be divided into three main groups. First of all there are the epidemiological studies in which the true number of RA-patients (both known and unknown) is established by means of population screening (e.g. the EPOZ survey). Secondly, there are health surveys in which, by means of questions posed to (selected) population groups, only those patients are identified among whom the disease has been diagnosed and who are themselves aware of the existence of the disorder - although this can readily lead to confusion with diagnoses of other rheumatic disorders. Thirdly, there are the general practice patient records, where again a selection has been made and only those patients seeking care are included. The patient group in question therefore varies according to the type of survey. This has significant consequences for the diagnosis-specific consumption. In this report, the survey method on the basis of which the data were collected is clearly indicated for each source of information.

For purposes of manageability the tables below have been broken down into five age groups (0-19, 20-44, 45-64, 65-79, 80+) and no distinction is drawn by sex. It has been decided to present the figures in the way in which they appear in the literature or were supplied by the institutions in question. The most important results are summarized in Chart 2.5 on pp. 142.

Before examining the consumption attributable to rheumatoid arthritis, it should be noted that some of the patients suffering from rheumatoid arthritis make little if any use of health care facilities. Although it is possible to criticize the survey method, the results of the CBS Health Interview Surve y (149) may, at the least, be regarded as striking. Of the 198 patients who indicated they were suffering from RA (i.e. osteoarthritis (chronic rheumatism, RA) of the hands or feet), no fewer than 37% turned out not to be receiving any treatment from a doctor for the condition. In addition over 50% of the RA-patients claimed that they had not used any anti-rheumatoid drugs during the past 12 months. A substantial proportion of the RA-patients therefore appears to make little if any use of health care facilities. The survey method employed, however, provides no assurance that all the individuals claiming to have RA do in fact suffer from the condition rather than other rheumatic disorders.

I Use of drugs

In the medicinal treatment of rheumatoid arthritis various drugs are used, prescribed either separately or in various combinations. In view of the hig hly individual nature of the symptoms and the risk of serious side-effects from the drugs, the prescription of medicines needs to be tailored as closel y as possible to the requirements of the individual patient. The choice of medicines is to a large extent determined by the symptoms. Other factors including the choice of drugs are the functioning of organs such as the liver, stomach and kidneys, the simultaneous use of other non-anti-rheumatic drugs and the proven effectiveness of the medication for the individual in question.

Anti-rheumatic drugs are administered by means of tablets, powders, suppositories or injections. The drugs may be divided into a number of groups depending on the aim they are designed to achieve (155, 156):

1. Pure painkillers for daily use (such as paracetamol and aspirin in low doses).

2. Fast-acting anti-inflammatory painkillers for daily use (aspirin and other NSAIDs).
3. Disease modifying anti-rheumatic drugs (DMARDs, such as anti-malaria drugs, gold compounds, penicillamine, sulphasalazine and cytostatics) and corticosteroids. These "second-line" drugs generally involve a greater risk of side-effects. Patients who use these drugs consequently need to be monitored frequently. The drugs only become effective after 3-6 months.
4. Drugs injected locally into or near an inflamed joint or tendon sheath (such as corticosteroids).

Quantitative data

A number of surveys are described below that provide information on the consumption of drugs by RA-patients. In interpreting the information below, the differences with respect to survey population and survey method need to be taken into account. A brief examination is also provided on medication compliance, the consumption of drugs for complaints due to side-effects of anti-rheumatic drugs, and self-medication.

Consumption of anti-rheumatic drugs:

Interesting figures emerge from the recently published findings on a study conducted by Leufkens et al. (157), in which the prevalence of RA in the population was estimated on the basis of the consumption of drugs. Over a two-year period (1987-1988) it was established among 29 pharmacists distributed throughout the Netherlands which patients had during this period:

- ever received a prescription for gold preparations or penicillamine, or
- received at least two prescriptions for NSAIDs and at least one prescription for an anti-malaria, sulphasalazine or cystostatics preparation, or
- had received at least two prescriptions for NSAIDs and had twice received corticosteroids, or
- had used long-term NSAIDs (> 180 days).

With respect to patients who satisfied one of the above criteria, the disorder(s) was then established by checking with the patient's general practitioner. A patient was classified by the GP as an RA-patient if the diagnosis had been definitively confirmed by a specialist. On the basis of these figures only 0.2% of the survey population could be classified as RA-patients. A number of explanations may be advanced for this (in comparison with other surveys) very low figure:

1. RA-patients being treated by alternative forms of medicine, administering self-medication or using a different type of drug were not identified.
2. The fact that general practitioners were used as the source of information in determining the prevalence is a possible source of underreporting, as it cannot simply be assumed that the general practitioner will be fully informed of all the disorders for which the patient is being treated by the specialist or will maintain a full record of all the details on the patient's health status.
3. RA-patients could be missed who are going through a stable period (or who fail to fetch the medication they have been prescribed) and who have not used any medication during the two survey years.

On the basis of this study it might cautiously be concluded that in view of the prevalence rates established in other studies, only a small proportion of the RA-patients use second-line medication (DMARDs, corticosteroids) or frequent NSAIDs. A substantial proportion of the RA-patients, therefore, appear not to use these drugs.

As part of the CBS Health Interview Survey (149), RA-patients were asked whether they had taken drugs for their disorder during the past 12 months. Approximately half (51%) replied in the affirmative (see Table 2.9). The fact that half the individuals claiming to have RA stated that they did not use any medicines for the disorder is a noteworthy finding. Once again, however, it is not established that all the individuals who claim to have RA did in fact suffer from the disorder.

In a very small-scale survey conducted among 23 RA-patients identified by means of enquiries among general practitioners, all the patients indicated that they used anti-rheumatic drugs. Virtually all the patients used both an NSAID and a DMARD. Some 13% of the patients interviewed indicated that they were also using an alternative drug at that point (158).

The results of a questionnaire submitted to 182 RA-patients receiving treatment in an outpatient rheumatology clinic (response rate over 90%) indicated that 87% used NSAIDs. Approximately 25% used anti-malaria drugs, 20% penicillamine and 5% were receiving gold treatment (152). The figures for NSAID use correspond well with those reported by the outpatient rheumatology department at the Leiden University Hospital, where some 75% of the RA-patients used an NSAID daily (159).

Table 2.9 Use of anti-rheumatic drugs over the past 12 months by RA-patients in 1989 (149)

Age	Sample size	Number of RA patients	Percentage of RA patients to have used an anti-rheumatic drug over the past 12 months*
0 - 19	2,262	3	53%
20 - 44	3,511	45	40%
45 - 64	1,775	79	53%
65 - 79	894	55	61%
80+	202	15	41%
Total	8,643	198	51%

* Percentages converted to reflect the composition of the Dutch population.

An interesting American study has been conducted on the basis of material supplied by California Medicaid (a health insurer for the less well-off) (160). Individuals have been classified as RA-patients in this study if they have made use of health facilities as a result of RA at least once during the survey year. The reason for use is given by the care provider. RA-patients not making any use of health care are not therefore represented in this study. On the basis of the claims submitted to the insurer in 1981 and 1982, over 75% of the RA-patients had received one or more prescriptions for NSAIDs on an annual basis. A quarter of the RA-patients had been prescribed steroid drugs (such as corticosteroids), while some 7% of the patients had been prescribed a DMARD (anti-malaria preparation, penicillamine). The majority of the latter group were also on NSAIDs. A very small proportion (2.6%) received gold injections. The extent to which US therapeutic policies correspond with the Netherlands, however, is unclear.

Compliance:
In a study conducted by Nienhuis (152) among RA-patients being treated at his own outpatient rheumatology department, 92% indicated that they were faithfully following their drug regimen. This may be regarded as a very high compliance rate, although it is possible that some of the patients were not prepared to tell their specialist that they were not keeping up with the treatment. After analysing 50 studies (not specifically relating to RA),

Blackwell (161) found a much lower patient compliance rate of 50-75%. The definition of the concept of compliance and the patient selection may help explain this discrepancy. Treatment compliance also depends on the kind of medicine. For aspirin and NSAIDs low compliances have been found in foreign studies (58-73%), and higher rates for DMARDs (83-84%) (162, 163).

Consumption as a result of side effects of anti-rheumatic drugs:
As indicated previously, anti-RA drugs can have iatrogenic complications. Ulcers in the stomach and small intestine, for example, are said to be 1.5-5 times more common among patients using NSAIDs (164). Dutch data on the excess uptake of medical care as a result of side-effects of anti-rheumatoid drugs are rare. The Californian study noted earlier (160) examined the use of drugs for gastro-duodenal disorders by RA-patients. This reveals that RA-patients receiving anti-rheumatic medication used far more drugs for gastro-duodenal disorders than RA-patients not using any anti-rheumatic drugs. This form of consumption is not generally attributed to RA, although it has in fact been a causal factor.

Self-medication:
By self-medication is meant the use of drugs not obtained on prescription. The CBS's Health Interview Survey (149) examined the application of self-medication in the previous 14 days. The findings showed that fewer than 1% of the RA-patients had used anti-rheumatic drugs without prescription over the past fortnight. This would suggest that RA-patients largely obtain their drugs through regular channels. Questions concerning the consumption of self-medication drugs against pain and fever (e.g aspirin) revealed that the percentage of RA-patients using these drugs was virtually equal to the proportion of non-RA-patients using them. The same applies to the general use of self-medication drugs (see Table 2.10).

A British survey conducted among 120 RA-patients being treated at four London hospitals (165), however, revealed that 54% of them regularly used simple analgesics. In nearly half the cases the consulting rheumatologist was unaware of this.

Table 2.10 Percentage of RA-patients and non-RA-patients to have self-medicated over the past 14 days (149)

Age	Sample size	Percentage to have applied self-medication*	
		RA patients (N = 198)	non-RA patients (N = 8,445)
0 - 19	2,262	0%	20%
20 - 44	3,511	39%	27%
45 - 64	1,775	23%	26%
65 - 79	894	21%	18%
80+	202	33%	17%
Total	8,643	26%	24%

* Percentages converted to reflect composition of Dutch population.

On the basis of above it may be concluded that:

1. Depending on the research background of the patient group, various patterns of medication were encountered.
2. Approximately three-quarters of RA-patients under specialist treatment use NSAIDs and some 25-50% (also) a second-line drug (DMARDs, corticosteroids).
3. In the studies in which the RA-patients were identified by means other than selection from hospital records, half the patients had used few if any drugs against RA.
4. There is considerable ambiguity about the extent of therapy compliance among RA-patients.
5. RA-patients who use anti-rheumatics make above average use of drugs for gastro-duodenal complaints.
6. Self-medication among RA-patients is not extremely high.

II Primary health care providers

General practitioners

In an average general practice of around 2,350 people, one to two diagnoses of RA will be made a year. Each general practice will have around 14 to 15 RA-patients, the severity and duration of whose illness will vary considerably (8).

The role of general practitioners in the care of RA-patients is the subject of considerable debate. Although the National General Practitioners Association (LHV) has not as yet issued an official statement concerning the treatment of RA, the LHV considers that the treatment of chronic diseases should initially be a matter for primary health care, with resort to secondary care in the event of exacerbations. Within the LHV it is generally expected that this rule of thumb will also be applied to rheumatoid arthritis. In 1985 the Netherlands Society of General Medical Practitioners wrote to the State Secretary of the Ministry of Health with respect to suggestions concerning rheumatology policy in which it indicated that the Society considered that most patients could be treated in the primary circuit (166).

If the general practitioner decides to refer a patient, this does not however mean that the former no longer plays a role of any significance. In the event of acute complications the general practitioner will often be the first person to deal with them. In addition, as family doctor, the general practitioner will play a significant part in helping the patient to come to terms with the disease, in helping the patient to fit the disorder and its consequences into daily life, in supporting the family and in organizing help, appliances and adaptations.

General practitioner care may broadly be divided into three elements: diagnostic, therapeutic and monitoring. The diagnostic function of the general practitioner in RA is examined briefly below. The actual role played by the general practitioner in the care of RA (also in relation to the specialist) is then examined, as well as the frequency of GP consultations.

Quantitative data

Diagnosis:
The diagnosis consists of taking down the case history and conducting a physical examination. Most rheumatologists would say that a proper diagnosis can only be made after specialist referral.

One study (111) has indicated that patients with undiagnosed RA consult their general practitioner for the following complaints/symptoms: complaints/-symptoms of the hand, fingers, wrist, leg, thigh, feet and toes. Unfortunately nothing is known about the specific measures then taken by the general practitioner.

Scope of general practitioner's role in relation to the specialist:
Various studies have described the actual division of roles between the general practitioner and the specialist in the care of RA. To some extent the differences in the research findings may be explained in terms of differences in the patient populations. The next section concerning referrals by general practitioners to other carers also provides information on the division of responsibilities between general practitioners and specialists.

The CBS Health Interview Survey (149) provides information on the role of the general practitioner in the care of RA-patients. Of the RA-patients, 27% indicated that the general practitioner was the main person they were consulting. Some 13% stated that they were being treated by both their general practitioner and a specialist, while approximately 23% of the patients reported that the specialist was their main therapist. The remainder, 37%, were receiving treatment from neither a general practitioner nor a specialist. These results are significant as they suggest that a comparatively high proportion of RA-patients regard their general practitioner as their principal or co-therapist. It should, however, be noted that the research group could include patients with rheumatic disorders other than RA.

The survey conducted among members of the Netherlands Rheumatism Association (109) also examines the role of the general practitioner in the care of RA-patients. Nearly 60% of the RA-patients turned out to have consulted their general practitioner during the survey year on account of the disorder (i.e. 40% had not) while 85% had consulted a rheumatologist. Respondents were also asked whom they regarded as the most important person in relation to the rheumatic disorder (no distinction was made in this respect in terms of specific rheumatic diagnostic groups). A fifth of the patients who had been in touch with a general practitioner in 1988 regarded the latter as the most important care provider. According to most respondents, the rheumatologist and physiotherapist played a much more important role. The general practitioner was particularly valued for the relationship of trust which the patient had with him/her.

A survey conducted among a sample of RA-patients drawn from the address lists of two rheumatology centres in Amsterdam and Groningen (64) revealed that at the time of the survey 95% of the patients were receiving specialist treatment for the disorder. From this it might be concluded that a maximum of 5% were being primarily treated by their general practitioner. On account of the way in which the patients were selected, however, these figures provide a distorted impression of reality. Nearly half the patients in the survey consulted not just a specialist but also their general practitioner for their RA, albeit less frequently. A notable finding from the study was that a higher proportion of patients from rural rather than urban areas consulted their general practitioner in connection with RA. A comparable study conducted in and around the town of Enschede similarly found that a higher proportion of patients in rural areas were in touch with their general practitioner than patients living in the city (110). In the survey conducted in and around Amsterdam and Groningen (64) patients were also asked whether they were satisfied with the interest taken in their condition by their GP. Nearly one third of the patients considered that their GP was not particularly interested in the full range of aspects to do with the disease.

A very small-scale survey (158) among 22 RA-patients whose names were obtained from a general practitioner revealed that 68% of the patients were in contact with their GP on account of the disorder (according to the patient and/or doctor). Some 95% had been in touch with a rheumatologist. Around 5% regarded their GP as the most important person they consulted, 23% regarded the GP as the coordinator of their treatment and 36% regarded the GP as providing support. Over 20% of the patients considered that the GP could improve the standard of care (e.g. by displaying greater interest and providing more information). In interpreting these findings allowance needs to be made for the fact that the data were derived from a very small number of patients and are not representative. Among other things the possibility cannot be excluded that precisely those patients were selected who consulted their GP frequently (for whatever reason).

To sum up, it may be concluded that the research findings concerning the size of the part played by general practitioners in the care of RA are often inconsistent. As noted earlier, the survey findings are heavily affected by differences in the research population and survey method. It is, consequently, impossible to make any clear statement concerning the role of the general practitioner in relation to the specialist. The survey findings discussed above indicate, however, that the general practitioner certainly plays a significant practical role in the treatment. According to the patients the general practitioner also plays a significant role as co-therapist, while some patients even regard their general practitioner as their main therapist.

Referrals:
A different kind of information providing insight into the measures taken by general practitioners in the treatment of RA-patients concerns referrals to different care-providers.

The clinical records kept by general practitioners affiliated to the NUHI (167) contain figures on referrals. The method of on-coding used is described in section 2.2.1.2. During the period 1971-1978, only 36% of all newly diagnosed RA-patients were referred to a specialist, 25% to a laboratory or X-ray department, 11% to other bodies (especially for physiotherapy) and 7% were admitted to hospital. A notable finding is the fact that the majority of the RA-patients were not referred to a specialist during this eight year period.

According to the Self-Sufficiency Project (111) conducted among persons aged 65 and over, GPs referred 14% of patients to other forms of primary care (especially physiotherapy) and 15% to secondary care (especially rheumatologists and internists) during RA consultations in the survey year. These referral percentages will in reality be much higher since some of the referrals will not have been included in the records (e.g. repeat referrals for patients under permanent treatment by a specialist may be made outside face-to-face contact).

The referral percentages found in the Transition Project (151) correspond closely with those in the Self-Sufficiency Project. In the Transition Project, 12% of the RA-patients were annually referred on account of the disorder to primary health care (95% to a physiotherapist) and 17% to a specialist (61% to a rheumatologist).

The Ommoord Monitoring Project (150) also provides information on referrals. On an annual basis 12% of the RA-patients were referred to a physiotherapist and 10% to a specialist for the first time.

In conclusion, the findings of the Self-Sufficiency Project, the Transition Project and the Ommoord Monitoring Project may be said to go in the same direction. In comparison, the results of the NUHI records differ sharply (i.e. fewer referrals per year). Apart from differences in the survey method, a possible explanation could be that individual general practitioners exert a major influence on the kind of care provided. The referral figures discussed above provide further support for the conclusion concerning the division of roles between the general practitioner and the specialist in RA care: once again, the part played by the GP in RA care turns out to be considerable.

Frequency of GP consultations:
Various sources of information are also available on the annual frequency of GP consultations by RA-patients. In the Self-Sufficiency Project (111) among persons aged 65 and older the average GP consultation frequency (as a result of RA) by RA-patients in the survey year was just under four per year. Notably, some 60% of the RA-patients consult their general practitioner only once or twice a year.

These figures may overreport the true situation, as the survey only covered patients who had in fact consulted their general practitioner on account of the disorder during the survey year. In calculating the average frequency of consultation, no account has therefore been taken of RA-patients who made no contact with their GP whatever.

A lower average frequency of GP consultation, namely 3.1 contacts on an annual basis, was encountered in the Transition Project (151), the survey method for which closely resembled that of the Self-Sufficiency Project. Once again a little over 60% of the RA-patients consulted their general practitioner only once or twice a year. The Transition Project related to the total practice populations (all ages) of the participating GPs.

Table 2.11 contains figures from the Ommoord Monitoring Project (150) concerning the average number of repeat consultations. The latter are defined as the average number of times that an RA-patient consults his or her GP in the course of a single year as a result of suffering from rheumatoid arthritis, having previously been in contact with the GP for the first time in the survey year as a result of RA complaints.

On the basis of the table it may be concluded that RA-patients who consulted their GP on account of the disorder did so on average 3-3.5 times a year.

Table 2.11 Average number of repeat GP consultations by RA-patients as a result of rheumatoid arthritis on an annual basis in 1979-1981 (150)

Diagnosis	Total number of consultations in two years	Number of repeat consultations on annual basis	
		year 1 (1979)	year 2 (1980)
Rheumatoid arthritis and related disorders*	490	2.0	2.4

* includes ankylosing spondylitis

From the survey conducted among members of the Netherlands Rheumatism Association (109) it emerged that RA-patients in contact with their general practitioner (59% of the total) had an average contact frequency (as a result of RA) of 8.6 on an annual basis. The average consultation frequency for all RA-patients was 5.1 per year.

As part of the "General Practitioners and Chronic Disorders" project conducted by the NIVEL in the context of its National Study (12), all consultations for a number of chronic disorders were recorded over a period of two years. The study was conducted in seven general practices (covering a total of 15 GPs). The research population totalled 23,500. The point-prevalence of RA in the research population was comparatively low, namely 58 patients or 0.25% (caused among other things by the youthful age structure of the population). The figures indicated that 19 RA-patients jointly consulted their general practitioner 20 times a year as a result of musculoskeletal problems. The remaining 39 patients had had no contact with their general practitioner during the survey period in connection with complaints of the musculoskeletal system. On average, therefore, RA-patients who consulted their general practitioner on account of such problems did so 1.05 times a year. Spread over all the 58 RA-patients the consultation frequency came to around 0.35 times per year.

The CBS Health Interview Survey (149) also provides information on the number of consultations of RA-patients as a result of RA. The reasons for medical consumption have been fairly broadly defined, namely rheumatism, joint discomfort, pain or trouble with limbs, etc.. House-calls, surgery appointments and telephone calls were all classed in the Health Interview Survey as consultations. In calculating the average consultation frequency the total number of consultations was divided by *all* respondents who indicated that they had rheumatoid arthritis. The figures therefore also include RA-patients who made no use whatever of health care facilities and patients receiving specialist treatment. In this way an average GP consultation frequency for all RA-patients of 1.7 per year was obtained (see Table 2.12). In view of the fact that the CBS Health Interview Survey indicated that some 40% of the RA-patients were being treated by their GP (as both main and co-therapist) the consultation frequency for this group of patients will have been around 4.25 per year.

Table 2.12 Average number of GP consultations by RA-patients as a result of rheumatoid arthritis, per RA-patient on annual basis in 1989 (149)

Age	Sample size	Number of RA-patients in sample	Consultation frequency per RA-patient*
0 - 19	2,262	3	-
20 - 44	3,511	45	1.0
45 - 64	1,775	79	1.3
65 - 79	894	55	2.7
80+	202	15	1.1
Total	8,643	198	1.7

* Multiplied by a memory factor and converted to reflect the composition of the Dutch population.

The results of the surveys concerning GP consultation frequency, as described above, do not entirely correspond. If all RA-patients are taken into consideration, an average annual GP contact frequency is obtained ranging from 0.35 to 5.1 (National Study and Rheumatism Association member survey respectively). These figures cover consultations as a result of RA or complaints of the musculoskeletal system. The variation in consultation frequency may in part be explained by differences in research method.

Medical consumption of RA-patients:
Given the very real possibility of underreporting of GP consumption attributable to RA in the above surveys (e.g. because RA-patients are more at risk of contracting respiratory infections, which will not however normally be recorded as consumption as a result of RA), the total consumption of RA-patients is examined below.

The Health Interview Survey of the CBS (149) makes it possible to compare the consumption of RA-patients with that of non-RA-patients.

Table 2.13 Total GP consultation frequency of RA-patients in comparison with non-RA-patients on an annual basis in 1989 (149)

Age	Size of CBS sample	Average number of RA-patients	GP consultations* non-RA-patients
0 - 19	2,262	4.29	2.92
20 - 44	3,511	9.00	3.19
45 - 64	1,775	8.33	3.68
65 - 79	894	8.20	5.30
80+	202	6.70	7.96
Total	8,643	8.60	3.61

* Multiplied by a memory factor and converted to reflect the composition of the Dutch population.

It may be seen from Table 2.13 that RA-patients have a higher GP consultation frequency on an annual basis than non-RA-patients (with the exception of the highest age bracket). The average difference is 5.0 contacts. From Table 2.12 and previous figures it is evident that roughly a third (1.7/5.0) of the extra consumption of RA-patients in relation to non-RA-patients may be explained by consumption as a result of RA. The remaining difference could be due to:

- underreporting of the consumption attributable to RA by the RA respondents;

- consumption as a result of other disorders encountered more frequently among RA-patients or which are apt to lead to troublesome complaints (and hence consumption).

To sum up, it may cautiously be concluded on the basis of the above that:

1. An average of 14-15 persons per general practice have RA.
2. Just how large a part the GP plays as consulting physician is unclear. The studies in this field are inconsistent. It may be concluded that GPs often act as co-practitioner and that some RA-patients even regard their GP as their main practitioner.
3. The average GP consultation frequency as a result of RA ranges in the various studies from 0.35 to 5.1 consultations per year per RA-patient.
4. If the number of GP consultations for the Netherlands as a whole as a result of RA is calculated on the basis of the prevalence as found by the NUHI (see Table 2.5) and the contact frequency as found in the CBS Health Interview Survey (1.7 and 5.0 respectively; see Tables 2.12 and 2.13), we arrive at a total of 159,000-467,000 per year.

Physiotherapists

Physiotherapy forms a significant part of the treatment of rheumatoid arthritis. Physiotherapy is used to preserve or improve muscle and joint function and prevent or correct deformities. It is also a significant factor in helping to reduce pain. Painful or stiff joints and muscles can react favourably to paraffin packs, hot baths, ice packs, ultrasound and electrotherapy or massage. Upon a reduction in pain active and passive exercises become easier (i.e. movement/remedial therapy). Passive movement (i.e. when the physiotherapist conducts the exercises for the patient) is aimed at maintaining the mobility of the muscles and joints and preventing stiffness. Active movement - including that against resistance - is mainly designed to improve mobility and build up muscle power.

Physiotherapy is always tailored to the needs of the particular individual. It is particularly important for the physiotherapist to train the RA-patient in a suitable programme of exercises at home, as the treatment will generally be continued at home by the patient by practising the exercises twice to three times a day for brief periods (168). Physiotherapy also plays an important role in regaining muscle power and coordination after a joint-replacement or other form of joint operation.

Apart from the medical side of the work, the nature of the profession and the comparatively high contact frequency mean that the physiotherapist generally also fulfils an important function in acceptance of the disease by the patient and making it part of daily life.

Treatment methods related to physiotherapy, from which RA-patients can benefit, are Mensendieck and Caesar therapy. These treatment methods are primarily geared towards correct posture and movement and the correct loading of the musculoskeletal system. This includes relaxation exercises to relieve pain. These may be taught by the physiotherapist, Mensendieck or Caesar therapist or be learned from yoga.

It is only fair to say that the research findings do not always provide an unqualified picture concerning the effects of physiotherapy in the treatment of RA (110, 152). In the survey conducted by Cornelissen (110), a number of rheumatoid patients indicated that the physiotherapy they had received had not been beneficial or that they had even been left worse off as a result of the tiring exercises/treatment or journey to visit the physiotherapist. Similarly the patient survey conducted by Nienhuis (152) indicated that 40% received only occasional or no benefit from the physiotherapy. Whether or not it is true that physiotherapy often has little or no effect or whether the research methodology left something to be desired is unclear. Certainly many individual RA-patients report positive experiences as well.

Quantitative data

An indication is provided below of the scale of the RA-patient group receiving physiotherapy and the total number of contacts in this respect.

Various sources suggest that the majority of RA-patients in outpatient treatment have received physiotherapy at some point: 76% (64), 66% (152).

Figures from a survey conducted in 1975 in a health centre in Rotterdam (169) indicate that of the 852 patients referred by the general practitioners to physiotherapists, 1% were referred as a result of rheumatoid arthritis. The CBS Health Interview Survey (covering 1986-1988) revealed that 11.5% of the Dutch population had had contact with a physiotherapist on an annual basis (170). Taking the two sets of figures it may roughly be calculated that over 17,000 RA-patients annually obtain physiotherapy (nearly 20% of the total number of RA-patients on the basis of NUHI figures (8)).

Other figures suggest that the number of RA-patients seeking physiotherapy is much lower than 20%. The Ommoord Monitoring Project (150), for example, indicated that only 12% of RA-patients were referred to a physiotherapist by their general practitioner on an annual basis. A similar figure - 11% - was found in the Transition Project (151) and the survey conducted by Meyboom-de Jong among persons aged 65 and over (111). An even lower referral figure of 4% was found in the "General Practitioners and Chronic Disorders" project conducted by the NIVEL as part of its National Study of Diseases and Treatments in General Practice (12).

Two other surveys, however, found higher percentages. In Rasker's survey (64) conducted among RA-patients nearly all of whom were receiving specialist treatment, a little over a quarter were receiving physiotherapy at the time of the survey. In particular, the more physically dependent patients resorted to physiotherapy.

The survey conducted among RA-patients of the Rheumatism Association (109) revealed that 55% had been in contact over the past year with a physiotherapist as a result of RA. The average contact frequency was weekly. The uptake of physiotherapy increased as bodily functioning deteriorated. Over one third of the rheumatoid patients interviewed who had contact with a physiotherapist regarded this person as their most important care provider. The most frequently cited reasons were the effects of the therapy in alleviating pain and preserving the suppleness of muscles and joints.

Of the RA-patients included in the survey, 56% confirmed that they had an exercise programme. On average the patients in question exercised 3.4 hours a week, spread over 5.5 days.

In Cornelissen's survey (110), 26% of the patients indicated that they were doing exercises at home prescribed by a physiotherapist. It was not asked whether the patients were still receiving physiotherapy treatment at the time of the survey.

In a survey conducted among his own patients, Nienhuis (152) recorded a much higher percentage of patients exercising at home, namely 82%.

The CBS Health Interview Survey (149) also provides information on the uptake of physiotherapy by RA-patients. Unfortunately the indication (diagnosis) for use is unknown. The figures therefore concern the uptake of physiotherapy by RA-patients (possibly but not necessarily as a result of rheumatoid arthritis) in comparison with the uptake by non-RA-patients. Table 2.14 indicates that RA-patients of all ages (with the exception of the 80+ age bracket) consulted a physiotherapist more frequently than non-RA-patients. If it is assumed that the two groups do not differ except for the fact that one group has RA, it may cautiously be concluded on the basis of Table 2.14 that some 30% of the RA-patients annually turn to physiotherapy on account of their disorder.

Table 2.14 Percentage of RA-patients and non-RA-patients to have visited a physiotherapist in the past year, irrespective of reason for contact, in 1989 (149)

Age	Size of sample	Percentage visiting pysiotherapist*	
		RA-patients (N = 198)	non-RA-patients (N = 8,445)
0 - 19	2,262	53%	4%
20 - 44	3,511	46%	13%
45 - 64	1,775	56%	18%
65 - 79	894	31%	18%
80+	202	7%	18%
Total	8,643	43%	12%

* Percentages converted to reflect composition of Dutch population.

Figures from the CBS Health Interview Survey (171) also indicated that patients with "rheumatic disorders of the joints" received some 25 physiotherapy treatments a year.

An important source of information in the future will be the NIVEL's Physiotherapy Surveillance Project. At present (1991) the project is still in the start-up phase. The intention is for 25-30 physiotherapists to act as monitoring stations. In addition data will be obtained from the general practitioners and patients concerned.

On the basis of the above it may cautiously be concluded that:

1. The effectiveness of physiotherapy in relation to RA is a matter of debate.

2. The majority of RA-patients have at some point received physiotherapy treatment (66-76%).
3. The number of RA-patients annually receiving physiotherapy for RA ranges in the various studies from 4% to 55%.
4. The average annual contact frequency of RA-patients receiving physiotherapy care varies in the surveys from 25 to 52 contacts.
5. A majority of the RA-patients (56-82%) say that they do exercises at home.

District nurse/health visitor

District nurses provide a wide range of care, with the aim of managing the disease and helping the patient to cope in family life and society. In the report "Suggestions for measures to combat rheumatism" issued by the National Home Nursing Association (1985), the responsibilities of district nursing in the care of rheumatism are listed as follows (172):

1. Nursing (physical hygiene care and nursing treatments).
2. Rehabilitation (promotion of physical health/strength, improvement of the physical environment, promotion of recreational opportunities).
3. Guidance and support for the patient and their home and work environment (coping, acceptance of the disease and the changing life-style).
4. Health promotion (provision of advice, identification of factors adversely affecting health).
5. Identification/instruction (identification of changes in the patient's situation, monitoring loss of functional capacity/use of appliances, instruction in the use of adaptations/appliances and encouragement of regular medical check-ups).

To sum up, the care therefore consists of the nursing of patients with highly disabling forms of rheumatoid arthritis, advising on the procurement of appliances and adaptations to the home, advice and support on coping with and accepting the disease and advice on claiming for expenses, etc. In addition the home nursing association has a stock of nursing items and appliances for temporary loan.

Apart from the overburdening of the district nursing service, the latter faces a number of other clear problems in the care it is able to provide to rheumatoid patients (172):

1. In many cases district nurses do not know enough about rheumatic disorders.
2. Rheumatoid patients are often unclear about what the district nursing service can and cannot do.
3. Patients generally find the succession of different district nurses annoying (as this cuts across continuity of care).
4. The division of responsibilities between the district nursing and home-help service is not clearly defined.

Area nurses play an important role in the tasks outlined earlier. An area nurse is a nurse working at regional or provincial level who concentrates on one or more areas, for example rheumatology care, and who has specialist nursing training in the area in question and special skills with respect to the transfer of knowledge. The National Home Nursing Association's report on rheumatic disorders referred to earlier (172) outlines the following tasks for area nurses:

1. Direct and indirect support to district nurses and health visitors and guidance and support for rheumatoid patients in the home environment.
2. Acting as a bridge and consultative link between hospital and non-hospital care providers and between various bodies.
3. Advising on facilities/adaptations and appliances.
4. Promoting the skills and expertise of district nurses and health visitors.
5. Provision of information and education (to patients and care providers).
6. Mediation in relation to the "individual help" provided by the Rheumatology Fund.

Among other things the ability to discharge these responsibilities depends on the availability of sufficient staff, expertise and skills, an adequate set of instruments and effective coordination with other carers in the RA field. Partly as a result of the reorganisations taking place in home nursing, there are at present numerous ambiguities about the future role of (rheumatology) area nurses.

Quantitative data

According to a survey conducted among 86 RA-patients (being treated by an outpatient rheumatology clinic) by the Twente Home Nursing Association (173), 33% stated that they were receiving district nursing care. There turned out to be a significant correlation between whether or not patients were receiving such care and Steinbröcker's functional classification (most RA-patients receiving district nursing care fell into the highest Steinbröcker categories (III and IV)). Of the RA-patients receiving such care, a fifth received help with bodily care. Among the majority of the patients the district nurse provided information on various aspects of the disorder (e.g. appliances, adaptations in the home, drugs, behavioural changes, self-help groups, the disease in general, coping with pain, preventive measures, and legal and financial regulations and arrangements).

Some 15% of the patients were seen by the district nurse daily or several times a week. Nearly three-quarters of the patients had a contact frequency of less than once a month. Around 60% of the patients were seen not just by the district nurse but also by the area nurse. At the time of the survey 5% of all respondents were receiving such care and 21% had received help from an area nurse over the past two years. Nearly all patients receiving district nursing care were satisfied with it.

Cornelissen's study (110) revealed that the uptake of district nursing care by RA-patients was five to six times higher than that of controls. In the case of the area nurse the uptake was as much as 8-9 times higher. Some 30-35% of the RA-patients interviewed stated that they were in contact with a district nurse each year. Around 10% of the rheumatoid patient respondents were visited by the area nurse. The average visit frequency of the district nurse was once a month, and of the area nurse several times a year. The contact with district nurses consisted primarily of guidance and support; actual nursing of those in need of care did not prove to be the most common task of district nurses.

The survey conducted among members of the Rheumatism Association (109) also examined the role of district nursing in rheumatology care. Of the RA-patients 22% indicated that they had been in contact with the district nursing service in the year preceding the survey. The average contact frequency of these patients on an annual basis was 33.5. Approximately 7% of the RA respondents (13 individuals only) indicated that they had been in touch with the area nurse. These patients indicated a strikingly high annual contact frequency: an average 17.6.

The survey conducted among RA-patients in Amsterdam and Groningen (64) indicated that 73% had never received help from the district nursing service. Some 17% were receiving such care at the time of the survey, while a further 10% were not receiving such care at that time but had done so earlier. The number of RA-patients receiving district nursing care varied in proportion with the degree of dependence.

Nearly 95% of the RA-patients interviewed reported that they had never received any help from the area nurse. Of the patients who had come into contact with this care provider, approximately half were still receiving home visits. The average contact frequency with this group was around six a year. The level of district or area nursing care varied considerably from region to region.

On the basis of the above it may cautiously be concluded that:

1. Approximately a quarter of the RA-patients annually turn to district nursing care, generally with a low contact frequency; the fact that a small proportion of the patients, however, have a very high contact frequency (daily or several times a week) means that an average contact frequency is obtained of around 34 on an annual basis.
2. District nursing care for RA-patients takes the form less of nursing than guidance and support.
3. The role of the area nurse varies from region to region. It may cautiously be concluded that on average 3-20% of the RA-patients are in annual contact with the area nursing service, with an average contact frequency of several to 18 a year (in all probability these are generally patients already receiving district nursing care).

Home-helps

The home-help service is designed to provide help to householders that are facing difficulties in managing their household tasks. Efforts are made to help the household to function independently. Where necessary the home-help service cooperates with other care providers, such as the district nursing service. Home-help activities fall into three broad categories:

1. Household tasks.
2. Caring tasks (including various forms of nursing).
3. Supportive tasks (psychosocial support, advice and support on tackling the household, education/care of children, etc.).

In the case of RA-patients, the care will generally take the form of advice and support for patients among whom the disease has been recently diagnosed and who require (temporary) support and advice on managing the household, and support for patients with serious, incapacitating forms of rheumatoid arthritis who are experiencing difficulties in coping with everyday activities as a result of the disorder.

Chronically ill rheumatoid patients making use of home-help are not always satisfied with this form of care. The booklet "Awkward patients are made" (174) sets out some of the problems and obstacles as experienced by RA-patients. Apart from organizational difficulties (many different home-helps, a change in the regular help after a number of years, unduly strict regulations concerning working hours and content of care, etc.), a lack of knowledge among home-helps concerning rheumatic disorders is also noted.

Quantitative data

The survey conducted among members of the Rheumatism Association (109) revealed that 31% of the RA-patients had received home-help in connection with the disorder during the survey year. The average annual contact frequency was 72.

The survey conducted among RA-patients receiving treatment at a rheumatology clinic (64) indicated that over three-quarters had never received home-help. Female and the more physically dependent RA-patients made more use than others of home-help.

Cornelissen's study (110) reveals that RA-patients had more paid household help than controls. This survey did not specifically examine the role of home-help, although it did reveal that roughly half the paid household help was subsidized, such as home-help, while the other half was paid for by the respondents themselves. Paid household help was more common in households in which the wife rather than the husband suffered from a rheumatic complaint.

On the basis of the above it may cautiously be concluded that:

1. Apart from official home-help, rheumatoid patients also obtain other forms of paid household help.
2. The extent to which use is made of home-help depends heavily on the sex of the patient and the severity of the disorder.
3. Annually approximately a quarter of RA-patients make use of home-help, with a contact frequency of 72 a year.

Social workers

The aim of General Social Work is the provision of information, advice and services as first port of call or longer term and/or systematic care to people and their environment in order to help prevent, reduce or solve difficulties arising from:

1. Disrupted or inadequate relationships between people and their social environment.
2. Coming to terms with events or circumstances affecting people's lives.
3. Inadequate basic conditions of existence.
4. Inability to cope and develop individually.
5. Unfamiliarity with regulations, facilities and other possibilities in society.

By definition social workers operate at the interface between individuals and their environment. The environment may consist of the primary community but may also cover public institutions such as hospitals and government agencies. In many cases social workers will work in harness with the core disciplines in primary health care, namely general practitioners, district nurses and home-helps (175).

Specific forms of assistance in the case of rheumatoid arthritis include psychosocial help in accepting the disease and fitting it into daily life and advice/mediation in practical problems such as applications for appliances/adaptations.

Quantitative data

Cornelissen's survey (110) reveals that RA-patients made use of social work 3-6 times more often than controls. Patients in urban areas made more use of social work than those in rural areas.

In the survey among members of the Rheumatism Association (109), 11% of RA-patients had come into contact with social work in the survey year. The average contact frequency on an annual basis was 5.4.

The survey conducted among RA-patients treated in an outpatient rheumatology clinic (64) revealed that 82% of them had never had any contact with social workers. At the time of the survey 7% of the patients were receiving visits from social workers from time to time (especially female and more dependent patients). The survey revealed once again that social work was more important in urban than in rural areas.

On the basis of the above it may cautiously be concluded that:

1. On an annual basis 7-11% of RA-patients come into contact with General Social Work, with an average contact frequency of around 5 contacts a year.
2. RA-patients who are female, have serious forms of RA and/or live in urban areas make more use of social work.

Alternative medical therapists

Patients consult alternative medical practitioners for highly varying reasons. These include lack of confidence in conventional medicine, dislike of conventional drugs, problems in the existing doctor/patient relationship and inability to accept an incurable disorder requiring lifelong treatment (medication), etc. In many cases alternative medical practitioners are consulted in addition to rather than instead of the orthodox practitioner (176). There are a great many different forms of alternative medicine such as homeopathy, acupuncture, anthroposophical medicine, manipulative therapy, health farms, enzyme therapy, nutrition therapy, etc.

The effectiveness of alternative forms of medicine is the subject of considerable debate. In an article Ter Riet (177) reached the conclusion that few controlled experiments had been conducted with a view to specifically examining the effectiveness of acupuncture in the treatment of RA. On account of the indifferent quality of the various surveys conducted in this field, the authors concluded that the effectiveness of acupuncture in the treatment of RA could not be taken as proven. Jacobs (178) conducted a survey of the literature in order to examine the effectiveness of alternative forms of treatment for patients with rheumatic disorders. He reached the conclusion that acupuncture, hydrotherapy, diets and dietary supplements, enzyme therapy, the green-lip mussel, homeopathy, manual therapy and feverfew had no more demonstrable therapeutic effect than control or placebo treatment.

A study conduced by Visser (179) revealed that nearly a quarter of rheumatologists themselves also (from time to time) prescribed one or more alternative forms of treatment (e.g. homeopathy, manual therapy and alternative diets). Even when the rheumatologist did not themselves use alternative forms of treatment the subject frequently came up in discussion with patients. Some 85% of the rheumatologists said that they spoke at least casually with patients about the possibilities/impossibilities of treatment by an alternative practitioner. Fewer than half (42%) of the rheumatologists advised patients one or more times a year to visit an alternative practitioner. Most rheumatologists did not have a favourable opinion about the effect of alternative medicine. Of the various forms of treatment, only health farms and manual therapy, acupuncture and homeopathy were somewhat more favourably viewed.

Quantitative data

Research findings by Cornelissen (110) reveal that RA-patients make more use of alternative practitioners than control individuals. Around 55% of RA-patients had at some point or other consulted an alternative practitioner. Among controls the figure was 22%. Most use was made of hands-on healers and homeopathy. Within the patient group there was a clearly discernible trend for patients to turn to alternative forms of treatment as their functional capacity declined. Further enquiry revealed that approximately half the patients experienced positive results (i.e. a reduction in complaints) from the alternative treatment.

In the survey among 182 RA-patients being treated by a rheumatologist (152), 31% indicated that they had tried alternative forms of medicine (homeopathy, acupuncture, magnetization and herbal therapy). Of these patients, only 23% said that the treatment had been beneficial.

In the survey on "rheumatic disorders and alternative forms of medicine" by Visser (179) noted above, 43% of the rheumatoid patients interviewed (among whom RA was the most common disorder) had at some point consulted an alternative practitioner for the disorder. Some 14% had gone to an alternative practitioner in the past year. The respondents indicated that they had made most use of spiritual healing, homeopathy and acupuncture. Over half those who had turned to alternative medicine discussed it with their rheumatologist (although generally not until they had actually visited the alternative practitioner).

The CBS Health Interview Survey (149) asked whether the respondent had been in touch with an alternative practitioner over the past year (see Table 2.15). The reason for the contact was not, however, established.

Table 2.15 Percentage of RA-patients and non-RA-patients to have had contact with an alternative practitioner over the past year irrespective of reason for contact, in 1989 (149)

Age	Sample size	Percentage to have had contact with an alternative practitioner*	
		RA-patients	non-RA-patients
0 - 19	2,262	47%	4%
20 - 44	3,511	16%	6%
45 - 64	1,775	18%	7%
65 - 79	894	12%	5%
80+	202	0%	2%
Total	8,643	15%	5%

* Percentages converted to reflect composition of Dutch population.

Table 2.5 indicates that more RA-patients than non-RA-patients turn to alternative practitioners in all age groups (with the exception of 80+). If it is assumed that apart from RA the two groups are otherwise identical, it may be concluded on the basis of Table 2.15 that some 10% of RA-patients annually consult an alternative practitioner for their disorder.

The survey conducted among members of the Rheumatism Association (109) also asked no questions about the reason for using alternative medicine. Over a quarter of the rheumatoid patients (not specifically RA-patients) indicated that they had been in touch with one or more alternative practitioners during the survey year (especially homeopathists, magnetizers and acupuncturists). Asked whether they had benefited from the treatment, 28% of the rheumatoid patients claimed to have had considerable benefit and some 60% no or only slight benefit.

It was suggested above that patients who fail to gain satisfaction from orthodox medicine may turn to alternative practitioners. The survey conducted among members of the Rheumatism Association (109) examined whether there was any correlation between satisfaction/dissatisfaction with professional carers and contacts with alternative practitioners. Notably, no such link was established. The survey conducted by Visser (179), however, indicated that 42% of those consulting an alternative practitioner did so because they were dissatisfied with their conventional treatment.

On the basis of the above it may cautiously be concluded that:

1. Despite the lack of persuasive data on the effectiveness of alternative forms of medicine, rheumatoid patients make considerable use of alternative forms of medicine.
2. One third to a half of the patients have at some point or another consulted an alternative practitioner for their disorder.
3. Those most frequently consulted were homeopathists, acupuncturists, magnetizers, hands-on healers, spiritual healers and herbal therapists.
4. On an annual basis some 10-25% of the patients turned to an alternative practitioner.
5. The use made of alternative medicine rises as functional capacity declines.
6. Approximately a quarter of the patients turning to alternative practitioners claim that the treatment is clearly beneficial.

II Care providers in secondary health care

Specialists

Various specialists are concerned in the outpatient care of RA-patients. Foremost among these is the rheumatologist (a doctor who has specialized in rheumatic disorders after several years of internal training).

Rheumatology has been formally recognized as a medical specialt in the Netherlands since 1948 and is on a comparatively small scale. The 110 or so rheumatologists working in the Netherlands account for 4% of the total number of internal specialists (180, 181). Converted in terms of the functional units referred to in the "Guidelines for the Hospital Facilities Act" there were around 84 functional units in 1989 (a functional unit is a measure of capacity for specialist work, corresponding with the average annual output of a specialist working full-time) (182).

Internists and pediatricians (the latter for the juvenile form of RA) are also important in the treatment of RA. As will be noted below, a proportion of RA-patients are in practice treated by an internist. Whether this is due to a shortage of rheumatologists so that RA-patients are "forced" to seek treatment from an internist or whether some RA-patients receive sufficient and adequate care from internists is not clear on the basis of the literature.

The actual division of responsibilities between general practitioners and specialists as the consulting physician for RA will not be examined further at this point; the subject was discussed in some detail in the section on GP care. In brief, it was concluded that a very high proportion of patients (ranging from 36% in the CBS Health Interview Survey (149) to 95% of the elderly participating in the Self-Sufficiency Project (109)) were being seen by a rheumatologist and that for some RA-patients general practitioners also fulfil the function of consulting or co-consulting physician (see pp. 103-105).

At this point is should be noted that the use of "second-line" drugs (e.g. anti-malaria and gold preparations and penicillamine) should preferably be handled by a rheumatologist in view of the knowledge and expertise required for their proper administration. Whether this is in fact the case, however, is unclear for lack of information.

Apart from the specialists noted above, orthopaedic surgeons, plastic surgeons, rehabilitation doctors, neurologists/neuro-surgeons, opthamologists and dermatologists play a part in the care of RA. They do not generally act as the primary therapist but are drawn in for the treatment of particular problems (e.g. complications, operations and joint replacements).

Pain clinics also play a part in RA care. Among other things they deal with the way in which pain is experienced, while techniques are taught for pain management. Among others anaesthetists and psychologists are involved in the treatment at pain clinics. For a number of years various hospitals in the Netherlands have employed specialized rheumatology nurses, consulting rheumatology nurses or community and hospital-based rheumatology nurses. These nursing staff generally work in outpatient clinics and deal especially with the more psychosocial implications of the disorder. Apart from helping the patient to come to terms with the disorder, rheumatology nurses also provide information on drugs and procedures for obtaining appliances and adaptations, etc. The rheumatology nurses are also designed to improve the continuity of care.

Finally it should be noted that the Netherlands Association of Rheumatologists considers the guideline on the permitted number of rheumatologists to be too low to provide an adequate standard of care now and in the future. A study is currently being conducted on behalf of the Ministry of Welfare,

Health and Cultural Affairs into the present and future requirement for rheumatologists if the demand is to be met.

Quantitative data

To begin with this section examines the division of responsibilities between the various specialists concerned with RA care. It also examines the share of RA-patients in the total patient population with rheumatic disorders in rheumatology practice. An indication is also provided of the average specialist consultation frequency.

Share of the various specialists in secondary health care:
The Health Care Information Centre (SIG) is in the process of setting up a system for recording outpatient treatments. No information is, however, as yet being collected, for which reason no reliable figures are at present available on the sharc of the various specialties in the treatment of RA-patients. Two surveys have however been conducted that provide a possible indication of the allocation of tasks.

Although the inpatient situation is not the same as the outpatient one, 55% of the patients admitted to hospital in 1986 with RA as the primary diagnosis (on the basis of SIG particulars) were treated by a rheumatologist. Internal medicine and orthopaedics both scored 18%, while at 4% and 3% respectively plastic surgery and paediatrics accounted for only a small proportion of the clinical care of RA-patients (181). It is however possible that these specialisms are regularly consulted by the rheumatologist or act as his co-practitioner.

The CBS Health Interview Survey also provides information on the division of roles between the various specialists in outpatient RA care (149). These figures indicate that the rheumatologist plays the greatest part in such care. Over 70% of the RA-patients in specialist care indicated that they were being treated by a rheumatologist. Only 5% were being treated by an internist and over 10% by an orthopaedic surgeon. It should however be noted that these figures are based on a very small number of patients.

Share of RA in total outpatient rheumatology care:
The Standard Diagnosis Surveillance of Rheumatic Disorders (SDR) is a largely outpatient surveillance system operated by the TNO Committee for Rheumatology Research. The monitoring project first got under way in a number of rheumatology practices in the Netherlands in 1978. Participation

is on a voluntary basis. In 1988 a total of 39 rheumatologists working in 20 practices participated in the SDR; in 1989 the figures had risen to 47 rheumatologists working in 21 practices. A number of practices only record the initial consultations (i.e. new patients); the remaining practices record all patients, i.e. both new and control patients. The SDR provides an insight into the share of RA-patients in the total patient population of the participating rheumatology clinics.

In 1988 an average of 11% of new patients (with a range of 3-26%) suffered from RA (i.e. definite, classical RA and RA with visceral or systematic disorders or Felty's syndrome). In 1989 the figure was 10% (range 2-31%). The average percentages among new and control patients combined in 1988 and 1989 were 33% (range 24-43%) and 24% (range 15-37%) respectively. The difference between 1988 and 1989 may be explained in terms of the fact that there were considerable changes in the group of participating rheumatologists, with a large practice with a low percentage of RA-patients participating in the monitoring project for the first time in 1989 (183, 184).

The widely differing percentages in the various practices is due to a number of causes, including the nature and composition of the practice, referral patterns, specific interests or expertise (resulting in a greater number of referrals) and the way in which criteria are applied, etc.

On the basis of the SDR, a rough estimate may be made of the absolute number of RA-patients being treated by a rheumatologist. In practices where all patients (i.e. new and controls) were recorded, 29 rheumatologists had some 6,300 RA-patients on their books in 1989. According to publications by the TNO Committee for Rheumatology Research (180) and the National Hospitals Institute (182), there were 111 rheumatologists working in the Netherlands in 1989, representing in total 84 functional units. In order to estimate the national total in 1989 the figure of 6,300 would need to be multiplied by a factor of 3, because the 29 rheumatologists participating in the monitoring project nearly all work full-time. This would then mean a total of nearly 19,000 RA-patients receiving specialist treatment from a rheumatologist in 1989.

It is not possible to use the SDR to obtain a fully reliable picture of the total uptake of specialist care by RA-patients because:

1. The monitoring project was not set up for this purpose.

2. The participating practices are not wholly representative of all rheumatology practices.
3. Not all rheumatologists participate in the SDR. The figures represent a third to a half of all rheumatologists.
4. The records do not contain figures on consultation frequency.
5. As other surveys have shown, RA outpatients are not all treated by rheumatologists but also by orthopedists, internists and paediatricians.

Consultation frequency:
Two kinds of specialist consultations may be distinguished. In check-up consultations the patient consults the specialist at regular, previously agreed intervals and the specialist checks the complaints and the use of medicines. In addition consultations take place at the patient's initiative in response to acute problems. The literature frequently stresses the importance of regular check-ups on the use of drugs with a substantial risk of side-effects. Little is however known about the actual extent to which RA-patients do re-consult specialists.

Few reliable data are available on the consultation frequency of RA-patients in specialist treatment. Figures issued by two rheumatology clinics provide some impression, although the clinics are not representative (one is established in a special rheumatology centre (the Jan van Bremen Institute) and one in a teaching hospital (Leiden)).

Approximately a fifth of the total number of patients in the rheumatology clinic at the Jan van Bremen Institute in Amsterdam consist of RA-patients. In 1989 there were between 2,500 and 3,000 RA-patients, with an average consultation frequency of nine a year. According to a spokesman for the Institute, this comparatively high consultation frequency may be explained because some of the RA-patients need frequent monitoring (as they use certain medicines) or regularly require an injection (e.g. of gold preparations) (185).

The Leiden University Hospital rheumatology clinic annually treats around 1,100 RA-patients (186). Some 50% of these RA-patients visit the clinic less than three to four times a year. The average consultation frequency is much lower than that in the Jan van Bremen Institute, averaging 4.6 a year (1988, 1989). A possible explanation for this difference may be derived from differing definitions of the concept of "consultation" or from different working methods in the two centres.

In Cornelissen's survey (110) the majority or RA-patients visited their rheumatologists at least once every three months (urban: 81%, rural: 64%). The difference between urban and rural patients may possibly be explained by the greater distance that rural patients have to travel in order to consult their rheumatologist. A related explanation is the fact that urban patients may regard visits to the laboratory (for check-up purposes) and attendance for injections as a specialist consultation. In contrast to the urban patients, rural patients generally turn to their general practitioner for these matters.

The survey conducted among members of the Rheumatism Association (109) also examined this question. The average consultation frequency among RA-patients who had visited a rheumatologist during the survey year was 6.7.

In the survey conducted among RA-patients by Rasker (64) half the RA-patients being treated by a rheumatologist visited the latter at least four times a year (some 15% even consulted the rheumatologist more than once a month) The other half had a lower contact frequency.

Figures on contact frequency may also be derived from material in the CBS Health Interview Survey (149). Table 2.16 indicates the average number of specialist consultations (nature of the specialism unknown) of RA-patients as a result of rheumatoid arthritis. The average consultation frequency per RA-patient has been calculated by dividing the total consumption among all persons who indicated they had RA, including those not receiving specialist treatment. From the table it may be seen that RA-patients consulted a specialist for their disorder on average one and a half times a year.

One of the findings of the CBS Health Interview Survey referred to earlier, however, was that only one third of the RA-patients are actually receiving specialist treatment. On this basis the average contact frequency of this patient group (irrespective of reason for contact) was 4.2 contacts a year.

In a number of years' time it will be possible to obtain a more reliable picture of the care provided to RA-patients by specialists when the Health Care Information Centre (SIG) will begin monitoring the number of outpatient specialist consultations (including reason for consultation) (the POLIS monitoring project).

Table 2.16 Average specialist consultation frequency per RA-patient as a result of rheumatoid arthritis on an annual basis in five age brackets in 1989 (149)

Age	Sample size	Number of RA-patients	Specialist consultation frequency per RA-patient*
0 - 19	2,262	3	0
20 - 44	3,511	45	1.13
45 - 64	1,755	79	2.17
65 - 79	894	55	1.57
80+	202	15	0
Total	8,643	198	1.52

* Multiplied by a memory factor and converted to reflect the composition of the Dutch population.

On the basis of the above it may be concluded that:

1. The rheumatologist is the most important of the specialists in hospital/-outpatient RA care (55-70%).
2. Of all initial consultations at rheumatology clinics an average of 10% are attributable to RA.
3. The share of RA in the total rheumatology practice (new and control consultations) amounts to around 25%.
4. A rough estimate indicates that approximately 19,000 RA-patients are receiving treatment by a rheumatologist.
5. The average contact frequency of RA-patients receiving specialist treatment in the surveys discussed varies. On the basis of figures supplied by the Leiden University Hospital, the surveys conducted by Cornelissen and Rasker and the CBS Health Interview Survey, an annual consultation frequency of 4.2 was found for the RA-patients receiving specialist treatment (from a rheumatologist).
6. If the specialist consultation frequency is calculated for all RA-patients, it may cautiously be concluded that the average annual consultation frequency is 1.5.
7. An estimate of the average number of specialist consultations for the Netherlands as a whole as a result of RA based on the prevalence as found by the NUHI (see Table 2.5) and the specialist consultation

frequency on the basis of the CBS Health Interview Survey (1.5 a year for all RA-patients) produces a figure of 140,000. According to figures supplied by the CBS (see page ...) 70% of the RA-patients receiving specialist treatment are being treated by a rheumatologist. Calculated for the Netherlands as a whole this means 98,000 annual contacts with a rheumatologist on account of RA.

8. If the total number of contacts in the Netherlands of RA-patients with a rheumatologist each year is made on the basis of the SDR figures on the number of patients being treated by a rheumatologist (19,000) and the average consultation frequency with rheumatologists calculated above (4.2), a figure of 80,000 contacts is obtained.

Ergotherapists

The aim of ergotherapy is to help support the patient to cope independently as effectively and as long as possible in his or her own home and work environment and to maximize the opportunities for self-reliance, productiveness and relaxation - in brief, to promote the activities of daily living (ADL).

A significant element of the ergotherapy instruction provided to RA-patients consists of teaching techniques for carrying out daily activities in such a way as not to place an unnecessary or incorrect load on the joints (such as getting up out of a chair, draining potatoes and putting on stockings).

Ergotherapy is tailored to the wishes of the individual concerned and to age, kind of handicap, living conditions, social circumstances, diagnosis and the anticipated progression of the disease. The ergotherapist is not just concerned with solving problems but also with preventing them. The ergotherapist can also play a significant role in applying for adaptations and appliances/facilities, ranging from special cutlery and chairs to vehicles and complete rehousing. In addition the ergotherapist can play a significant part in helping the patient to accept and make effective use of new facilities. In many cases, acceptance of an appliance means crossing a "psychological threshold" by the patient, in which the ergotherapist can play a significant part.

At present, however, it is difficult for patients to obtain ergotherapy. On account of financial stringency, ergotherapy can in general only be obtained from institutions (e.g. nursing homes, rehabilitation clinics and hospitals). It is rarely provided on an outpatient basis; it can only be provided on a non-hospital basis as part of the day-treatment provided in nursing homes and rehabilitation clinics. Ergotherapy is also being provided in primary care on an experimental basis in a limited number of places in the Netherlands (187, 188).

Although the additional travel time would involve an increase in the workload, research suggests that it would be useful to extend ergotherapy to primary health care, especially in the home situation (187, 188). The carer would then be dealing with the day-to-day environment faced by the patient. On this basis the ergotherapist would be able to give more precisely tailored advice, so that the patient would be able to cope more effectively and to remain as independent as possible.

Quantitative data

The survey conducted among RA-patients by Rasker (64) indicated that 70% had never had any contact with an ergotherapist. The remaining 30% who had had such contact were virtually all from the greater Amsterdam area. In particular this is attributable to working methods at the Jan van Bremen Institute, where the RA-patients were under treatment.

In the survey conducted among the members of the Rheumatism Association (109), 15% of the RA-patients indicated that they had been in touch with an ergotherapist in 1988. In that year these patients had had an average of 15 contacts with this carer.

On the basis of the above it may cautiously be concluded that:

1. In view of the financial stringency surrounding ergotherapy, not many RA-patients are able to draw on this kind of care.
2. On an annual basis some 15% of RA-patients consult an ergotherapist, with an average of 15 contacts.

III Secondary health care organizations

Hospital

RA-patients may be admitted to hospital for various reasons, for example when the disease cannot be controlled by outpatient treatment and it is necessary to switch to using drugs which are so aggressive that there is a risk of serious side-effects, or when surgery is necessary to reduce pain or restore function, or where symptoms arise (e.g. as a result of complications) which necessitate hospital treatment. The care provided in general hospitals concentrates primarily on the somatic aspects of the disease, while specialized rheumatology hospitals and rehabilitation centres cover a much broader field.

Quantitative data

A national register of day admissions is kept by the Health Care Information Centre (SIG) (National Medical Registration System) (189). In 1989 76 hospitals took part in the day-care surveillance project. Since no information is available on how many hospitals have day-care facilities, however, it is unclear whether the figures obtained from these records present a complete picture: if some hospitals with day-care facilities did not participate in the project, the figures will not reflect the total consumption of these facilities. According to the register, 56 patients were admitted to day-care in 1989 as a result of RA (excluding juvenile RA). Of these, 41% underwent surgery (this compares with 30% of patients who were admitted for hospitalization, see Table 2.17). As the table shows, a relatively large number of patients were admitted to day-care as a result of RA in 1989 compared with other years (1986: 26 admitted to 54 hospitals; 1987: 27 in 64 hospitals; 1988: 20 in 76 hospitals; 1989: 56 in 76 hospitals).

The SIG includes virtually every hospital in the country in its register of hospital admissions (99.5% in 1989). Two centres which are important for rheumatic disease, namely the Beatrixoord in Haren and the St. Maartenskliniek in Nijmegen, took part in the surveillance project; however, since the National Medical Registration System ignores specialized institutions catering for patients requiring lengthy treatment, RA-patients admitted to the Beatrixoord, in contrast to those admitted to the St. Maartenskliniek, are not included in the statistical summaries produced by the Registration System. Two other important rheumatology hospitals did not take part in the project, namely the Daniël den Hoed hospital in Rotterdam and the Sole Mio in Noordwijk aan Zee. This should be taken into account when interpreting the figures in the table.

Table 2.17 shows the number of admissions and hospital days as a result of rheumatoid arthritis, analyzed by ICD code (189).

Table 2.17 Absolute number of hospital admissions and hospital days, average length of stay, percentage emergency admissions, patients undergoing surgery in 1989 for RA in the Netherlands (*) and number of admissions for RA as primary and secondary diagnosis together (189)

ICD code	Number of admissions	Percentage distribution	number of hospital days	Average length of stay (days)	Emergency admissions (%)	Underwent surgery (%)	Admissions: RA as primary + secondary diagnosis
714.0 Rheumatoid arthritis	4,112	99.4	96,751	23.5	16	30	8,222
714.1 Felty's syndrome	18	0.4	556	30.9	67	6	39
714.2 Other forms of RA, visceral, generalized	7	0.2	148	21.1	43	14	23
RA	4,137	100	97,455	23.6	16	30	8,284

* Excluding Beatrixoord, Daniël den Hoed and Sole Mio, among others.

It can be seen from the Table 2.17 that there were more than 4,100 admissions in 1989 for RA as primary diagnosis (RA-ICD-codes: 714.0, 714.1 and 714.2), involving a total of approximately 97,500 hospital days. More than 99% of the admissions resulting from RA were registered under code 714.0 "rheumatoid arthritis". In his commentary on the SIG-data (190), the rheumatologist Cats expresses surprise at this fact, since in his opinion RA-patients are usually admitted as a result of generalized symptoms or visceral disorders (code 714.2). It is extremely likely therefore that there is a registration problem here.

The average duration of each RA-admission was approximately 24 days. Less than a fifth of these were emergency admissions. Almost a third of the patients underwent surgery during their hospital stay, the most common operations being arthroplastic surgery on the knee and hip joints and synovectomies (190).

In order to estimate the total number of admissions and hospital days in the Netherlands resulting from RA, data are needed from the two rheumatology hospitals not included in the SIG-register. The rheumatology department of the Daniël den Hoed clinic admitted approximately 160 patients in 1989 as a result of rheumatic disease (no differentiation into different diagnosis categories), with a total of 16,356 hospital days. The average hospitalization period was 24.8 days (191). In Sole Mio, 244 patients with joint disorders were admitted in 1989. In 197 of these cases (81%) the admission was as a result of RA. The total number of hospital days for patients with joint disorders was 12,993, and the average length of stay in that year was high at 53.3 days (no differentiation into diagnosis categories). Surgery was indicated (192) for 34 RA-patients (17%).

The total number of admissions as a result of RA in the Netherlands as a whole is estimated at almost 4,900 per annum, and the number of hospital days at over 121,000. These figures are based on the assumption that in both the Daniël den Hoed and Sole Mio 80% of the admissions and hospital days were due to RA.

According to the SIG-data, in addition to the 4,000-plus admissions resulting from RA (Table 2.17) in 1989, there was a similar number of admissions in which RA was reported as a secondary diagnosis. It is highly possible that some of these admissions were the result of RA, particularly surgical admissions (orthopaedic and plastic surgery), where the causal disorder may not always be stated as the primary diagnosis. The number of admissions to which this might apply, however, is not known.

Approximately 55% of the admissions as a result of RA (primary diagnosis) in 1986 were in rheumatology departments; 18% of patients were admitted to internal medicine departments, and a further 18% to orthopaedic departments. The remaining 9% were treated in a variety of departments, including plastic surgery, paediatric, surgical and neurological units (193). In 1987 305 hospital beds were occupied in the Netherlands as a result of RA (189).

Table 2.18 shows the number of hospital admissions and hospital days with RA as primary diagnosis (ICD-codes 714.0 to 714.2 inclusive) for five age categories (189).

Table 2.18 Absolute number of admissions, hospital days and average length of stay in hospitals resulting from rheumatoid arthritis for five age categories, 1986 (189)*

Age	Number of hospital admissions	%	Number of hospital days	Average length of stay
0 - 19	34	(0.8)	1,351	39.7
20 - 44	446	(11)	9,242	20.7
45 - 64	1,656	(41)	43,406	26.2
65 - 79	1,665	(41)	50,996	30.6
80+	264	(6)	9,018	34.2
Total	4,065	(100)	114,013	28.0

* Number of hospitals taking part in the surveillance project was 99.1% in 1986 (figures exclude Beatrixoord, Daniël den Hoed and Sole Mio, among others).

It is apparent from the table that people in the age range 45-80 place the greatest demand on hospital facilities (more than 80% of the admissions resulting from RA). The average length of stay was 28 days in 1986 and fluctuated widely between the different age groups (high in the youngest age category and low in the category 20-45). There was a sharp fall in the average length of stay in the period between 1983 and 1989, from 33 days per admission in 1983 to 24 days in 1989 (190). The number of admissions resulting from RA increased in the same period from 3,817 in 1983 to 4,137 in 1989. When adjusted for the percentage of hospitals which took part in the surveillance project, this represents an increase in the number of admissions of 6.2%.

The SIG-data presented in the table give no information about the consumption of hospital facilities per RA-patient, however. One source from which this consumption can be related directly to the RA-patient group is the study carried out among the members of the Rheumatism Association

(109). This survey asked whether respondents had ever been admitted to hospital as a result of their rheumatic disease. Approximately 70% of the RA-patients confirmed that they had been admitted to hospital at some time. On average, members of this group had been admitted 3.8 times for a total of 97 days per patient (approximately 36 days on average per admission). Information was also sought about operations carried out in connection with rheumatic disease. Unfortunately, the description of the results did not indicate what proportion of the RA-patients had undergone surgery, though it was stated that the majority of operations for rheumatoid arthritis had been carried out on knees, hands, hips and feet.

The CBS Health Interview Survey (149) asked about the number of hospital admissions (and the reason) in the year preceding the survey (see Table 2.19). The findings showed that of every 1,000 RA-patients, 40 were admitted to hospital each year as a result of rheumatoid arthritis. It should be borne in mind here, however, that the sample size in the Survey (N = approx. 8,500) is rather small for an estimate of consumption of hospital facilities, and a degree of caution should therefore be exercised in interpreting the results.

Table 2.19 Number of hospital admissions as a result of RA per 1,000 RA-patients in five age categories on an annual basis, 1989 (149)

Age	Sample size	Number of RA-patients in sample	Admission frequency per 1,000 RA-patients*
0 - 19	2,262	3	0
20 - 44	3,511	45	60
45 - 64	1,775	79	20
65 - 79	894	55	60
80+	202	15	0
Total	8,643	198	40

* Frequencies converted to the Dutch population structure and composition

On the basis of the above, it may cautiously be concluded that:

1. A sizeable proportion of RA-patients have been admitted to hospital at some stage in connection with RA.

2. Of every 1,000 RA-patients, approximately 40 are admitted to hospital each year in connection with their disease.
3. In 1989 there were almost 4,900 hospital admissions as a result of RA, involving a total of over 121,000 hospital days; in addition, RA was stated as a secondary diagnosis in approximately 4,000 other admissions.
4. More than three-quarters of admissions involved patients aged between 45 and 80.

IV Tertiary care organizations

(Rheumatic) rehabilitation centres

Rehabilitation may take place after an acute phase of a disease, accident or surgical operation. The purpose of the treatment is to prevent restrictions and handicaps or to influence these in such a way that the patient is able to attain optimum function given his or her capacities and circumstances.

Rheumatology patients, usually suffering from a combination of somatic, psychological, social and/or relationship problems, receive specialized rehabilitation treatment in rheumatology rehabilitation centres. The rehabilitation process is determined by the efforts and participation of the patient. The treatment is team-based (multidisciplinary), under the leadership of a rehabilitation physician, and may be hospital-based or provided on an outpatient basis.

There are several rheumatology centres in the Netherlands which provide rehabilitation treatment to a greater or lesser extent, namely the Beatrixoord in Haren, the St. Maartenskliniek (Nijmegen), Sole Mio (Noordwijk aan Zee), Daniël den Hoed (Rotterdam) and the Jan van Bremen Instituut (Amsterdam) - though officially only the Beatrixoord and the St. Maartenskliniek are recognized as rheumatology rehabilitation centres. Rehabilitation treatment is not only provided in specialized rehabilitation centres, however, but also in hospitals and nursing homes.

Quantitative data

In the survey of members of the Rheumatism Association (109), 14% of the RA-patients stated that they had been admitted to a (rheumatology) rehabilitation centre at some time, the average number of admissions being two. 35% stated that they had undergone rehabilitation treatment. The SIG is collecting information nationally regarding the number of admissions and nursing days/appointments at rehabilitation centres (REVIS-surveillance project (194)). The figures stated below relate only to a small proportion of all admissions for RA to rheumatology rehabilitation centres, i.e. those in which the *rehabilitation physician* carried out the admission. In 1986 ten of the 22 rehabilitation centres took part in the surveillance project, including two centres which are important for rheumatic disease, the St. Maartenskliniek and the Beatrixoord.

The medical consumption of RA-patients admitted for rehabilitation has largely been incorporated in the figures presented on the foregoing pages dealing with hospital care. In this section separate attention will be given to the uptake only in the case of admissions by a rehabilitation physician.

The REVIS project shows that in the ten participating centres, 26 patients were admitted in 1986 *by rehabilitation physicians* with RA as the primary diagnosis, with a total of 3,100 nursing days. This represented 0.78% of all patients admitted to rehabilitation centres and 0.89% of all nursing days. If RA as a secondary diagnosis is also included in the calculations, it emerges that a total of 48 RA-patients were admitted by rehabilitation physicians in the rehabilitation centres taking part in the REVIS-project, with a total of 5,200 nursing days. Only five rehabilitation centres took part in the monitoring of outpatient treatment and, since it is not known how many rehabilitation centres have outpatient facilities, it is not possible to say anything about the coverage of the REVIS-project. The rehabilitation physicians from the five participating centres reported 64 patients in 1986 who were receiving outpatient treatment as a result of RA (as primary diagnosis), with a total of more than 2,000 visits. RA as a secondary diagnosis was relevant in only five patients who had been admitted for outpatient care by rehabilitation physicians (194).

On the basis of the above, it may cautiously be concluded that:

1. A not insignificant proportion of RA-patients state that they have undergone rehabilitation treatment at some time as a result of their disease.
2. It is striking that rehabilitation physicians admit more RA-patients for outpatient care than for hospital treatment.

3. At least 26 RA-patients per year are admitted to rehabilitation centres by rehabilitation physicians on account of their disease; they account for at least 3,100 nursing days at these centres.

Nursing homes

Like the rehabilitation centres, nursing homes are usually divided into those providing outpatient care and those providing a full nursing service. Outpatient treatment, which involves the patient remaining at the nursing home for a day or part of a day, can avoid the need for an admission, or can shorten the duration of such an admission. A distinction is made according to the nature of the treatment or nursing given, into somatic and psychogeriatric treatment.

Patients are often admitted to or treated in nursing homes for a combination of reasons; in addition to practical reasons, there are often several disorders involved. The tables below are therefore not based on the number of admissions or treatments in nursing homes where RA was stated as the first (main) diagnosis, but are based instead on the number of admissions or treatments where RA was stated as the first, second or third diagnosis.

Patients can be admitted to a nursing home for reactivation or for an indefinite period. In discussions with experts it repeatedly emerges that nursing homes sometimes function as temporary reception centres for RA-patients, who are admitted to the nursing home for a period of several weeks in order to relieve the overburdened informal care network surrounding them, or enable the carers to take a holiday, etc.

There is one nursing home in the Netherlands which specializes in providing nursing care and treatment for patients with the most severe form of RA, namely the Rheumaverpleeghuis in Rotterdam, which has 46 beds. Nursing care and treatment are provided by a multidisciplinary team, and two consultant rheumatologists are attached to the nursing home.

Quantitative data

The SIG (SIVIS-surveillance project) has numerical data on the reasons for admission to the nursing homes. In 1988 82.7% of the nursing homes took part in this project. Information was recorded both at the start and at the end of the admission, as well as on a reference date (13 September). On the basis of the first three admission diagnoses, RA is more frequently recorded as the first diagnosis in somatic departments, and more frequently as the second or third diagnosis in psychogeriatric departments.

According to the SIVIS-register (195) approximately 130 patients were admitted for outpatient treatment in 1988 as a result of RA, with a total of approximately 3,900 treatments being given (see Table 2.20). The number of treatments per patient averaged 30. The share of rheumatoid arthritis (as one of the first three admission diagnoses) in the total number of admissions for outpatient treatment was 3.4% in somatic departments and 0.7% in psychogeriatric departments.

In 1988 more than 400 patients were admitted to nursing departments with RA as one of the first three admission diagnoses. The average length of stay was approximately 537 days. The share of RA (as one of the first three admission diagnoses) in the total number of admissions to nursing homes was 2.7% in somatic departments and 0.7% in psychogeriatric departments.

Table 2.20 Number of patients admitted for *outpatient treatment* with RA as one of the first three admission diagnoses, and total number of treatments for three age categories, 1988 (195)*

	Somatic		Psychogeriatric	
	Number of admissions	Number of treatment days	Number of admissions	Number of treatment days
0 - 64	13	461	2	103
65 - 79	59	1,552	5	324
80+	43	1,189	8	254
Total	115	3,202	15	681

* Participation rate = 82.7%

In order to obtain an accurate picture of the annual uptake of care by RA-patients, Table 2.21, given the average length of nursing care (more than one year), is based on the data obtained on the reference date. On this date there were approximately 825 persons in nursing homes with RA as one of the first three admission diagnoses, involving a total of more than 300,000 nursing days in 1988.

The SIVIS-register also records the help index for all patients admitted or treated. This index gives an insight into the need for care. Data taken from the SIVIS-register showed that the help index for RA-patients did not differ greatly from the usual help index for patients admitted to nursing homes.

Table 2.21 Number of patients admitted to the nursing department in *nursing homes* on the reference date with RA as one of the first three admission diagnoses, and the number of nursing days for three age categories, 1988 (195)*

	Somatic		Psychogeriatric	
	Number of patients on ref. date	Number of hospital days	Number of patients on ref. date	Number of hospital days
0 - 64	46	16,790	2	730
65 - 79	294	107,310	29	10,585
80+	366	133,590	88	32,120
Total	706	257,690	119	43,435

* Participation rate = 82.7%

On the basis of the above, it may cautiously be concluded that:

1. Converted for the Netherlands, almost 160 patients with RA as one of the first three admission diagnoses are admitted for outpatient treatment annually, involving a total of more than 4,500 treatment days.
2. Converted for the Netherlands, almost 1,000 patients with RA as one of the first three admissions diagnoses are in a nursing home, involving a total of more than 360,000 nursing days per year.

2.2.4.3 Conclusion

This section has presented a large number of figures relating to the demand placed on the care system as a result of rheumatoid arthritis. The findings relating to the various forms of care are summarized on the following pages (see Chart 2.5). It should be stressed once again at this point that it is highly likely that the picture painted here underestimates the true uptake of care facilities as a result of RA.

Chart 2.5 Summary of the main findings regarding uptake of care as a result of RA

Drugs	- More than three-quarters of the RA-patients being treated by specialists use NSAIDs, and approximately 25-50% (also) use DMARDs (secondary medication); - In the studies consulted where the RA-patients were obtained other than by selection from the files of a(n) (outpatient) clinic, approximately half the patients use little or no medication to treat rheumatic disease; - Self-medication by RA-patients is not common;
General practitioners	- The true extent of the role played by GPs in providing treatment is unclear, since the findings of studies in this field are extremely diverse. It can be concluded that the general practitioner often acts as a co-therapist, and that some patients even regard their GP as the main therapist; - The average number of consultations with the general practitioner as a result of RA varies in the different studies from 0.35 to 5.1 consultation per RA-patient per year; - If the number of consultations with GPs as a result of RA is calculated for the Netherlands as a whole, a figure of between 159,000 and 465,000 contacts per year is found;

Physiotherapists

- The number of RA-patients per year receiving treatment from a physiotherapist because of RA ranges in the studies from 4% to 55%;
- The average annual contact frequency of RA-patients under the care of a physiotherapist varies from 25 to 52 contacts;

District nurses

- District nursing care for RA-patients focuses less on actual nursing care and more on guidance and support;
- Approximately a quarter of RA-patients use the district nursing service each year, with an average contact frequency of around 34 contacts;
- Depending on the study findings consulted, between approx. 3% and 20% of RA-patients have contact with an area nurse each year, with the average contact frequency ranging from a few to 18 contacts;

Home helps

- The extent to which the home help services are called on is influenced by the sex of the patient;
- Approximately a quarter of RA-patients call on the home help service each year, with a contact frequency of approximately 72 contacts per annum;

Social workers

- On an annual basis between 7% and 11% of RA-patients have contact with the general social work service, with an average contact frequency of approx. 5 contacts per year;

Alternative therapists

- Between a third and half of RA-patients have had contact with an alternative therapist at some time because of the disease;
- Approx. 10%-25% of RA-patients are treated by an alternative therapist each year;

Specialists

- As regards other specialists, the rheumatologist is quantitatively the most important figure within the in-patient/outpatient RA-care system;
- 10% of all initial consultations at rheumatology clinics take place as a result of RA; the percentage of all consultations (both new and follow-ups) is around 25%;

- Around 19,000 RA-patients are being treated by a rheumatologist;
- The majority of RA-patients being treated by a specialist consult him/her around 4.2 times a year;
- Calculated for all RA-patients, an average annual specialist consultation frequency of 1.5 is obtained;
- The annual number of specialist consultations as a result of RA is estimated at at least 140,000 for the Netherlands as a whole, between 80,000 and 98,000 of which are with a rheumatologist.

Ergotherapists

- The financial constraints on occupational therapy mean that few RA-patients are able to make use of this type of care;
- On an annual basis approximately 15% of RA-patients receive ergotherapy, with an average total of 15 contacts;

Hospitals

- Approximately 40 out of every 1,000 RA-patients are admitted annually as a result of the disease;
- In 1989 there were 4,900 hospital admissions with RA as the first admission diagnosis, involving a total of more than 121,000 hospital days;

(Rheumatology) rehabilitation centres

- A not insignificant proportion of the RA-patients have received rehabilitation treatment because of the disease;

Nursing homes

- Almost 160 patients with RA as one of the first three admission diagnoses are admitted for out-patient treatment annually, involving a total of more than 4,500 treatment days;
- Almost 1,000 patients with RA as one of the first three admission diagnoses stay in a nursing home annually, involving a total of more than 360,000 nursing days.

2.3 Comparison with other countries

2.3.1 Occurrence of RA

There are indications of international variation in the **prevalence** of RA among the population. The prevalence of definite RA (see Annex 2) is in the region of 1% to 2% in the majority of white population groups (48). Among African negroes, by contrast, a low prevalence of 0.1% is found (196), while the prevalence among North American Indians is approximately 6% (197, 198). The findings of surveys carried out in a number of Northern European countries also point to a higher prevalence: 3% in Heinola, Finland and 5% in Oberhölen in Germany (200). On the basis of data taken from the EPOZ (see section 2.2.1) it can be concluded that the Netherlands occupies a mid-position, with a prevalence which corresponds to that found in the majority of white population groups (approximately 1-2%).

There is also clear international correspondence in terms of age and sex-specificity, with the prevalence among women always being two to three times higher than among men, and increasing with age for both men and women (48).

When comparing several different studies, however, it is important to consider to what extent observed variations in prevalence can be attributed to differences in study methods, including differences in diagnosis, and how far they are due to genuine variation (in immunogenetic predisposition and exposure to primary causal factors; see section 2.2.1.4). It is difficult to make any firm statements about this at the moment.

As described earlier, the prevalence of RA is the result of inflow and outflow of patients. The inflow is the incidence, while the outflow is the sum of remission and lethality (Figure 2.2). No figures are available for the Netherlands on **remission** which would enable a comparison with other countries to be made. The level of remission indicated by the findings of a few studies is described in section 2.2.1.3.

International data on the **incidence** of RA are scarce. This is in part due to the fact that in order to determine incidence it is necessary to study a large population over a period of many years. Where data are available, they are only comparable to a limited extent since they are often based on differing diagnostic criteria. In those cases where the same ARA criteria of 1958 have been used (3), the incidence of RA in the Netherlands (9) corresponds with that in Japan (49) at approximately 1/1,000, while the incidence in Massachussets is higher at 3/1,000 (201). A rough general estimate would be that the international incidence is around 1/1,000 on the basis of the ARA criteria.

As indicated in section 2.2.1.3, data on mortality taken from death certificates are too unreliable to provide any insight into the outflow from the RA-population as a result of death. Comparison with the stated cause of death is also of limited use due to international differences in clinical practice (differences in the diagnosis and registration of RA) and differences in registration (of primary and secondary causes of death) on the death certificate.

Another way of measuring the outflow from the RA-population as a result of lethality is to look at data on the reduction in life expectancy in patients with RA compared with the population as a whole (see section 2.2.1.3). With the occasional exception, it can be concluded on the basis of several studies that, internationally, there is a reduction in the life expectancy of RA-patients in relation to the general population. The length in years of this reduction in life expectancy is unclear, however, due to differences in study methods (including differences in diagnostic criteria, differences in patient selection (hospital, open population), and differences in the length of the follow-up period).

It can be **concluded** that differences in study methods and in the diagnostic criteria used rule out firm statements regarding the international differences found in the epidemiological parameters of RA. It would appear, however, that the Netherlands occupies an intermediate position internationally with respect to the prevalence of RA.

2.3.2 Articular features and extra-articular manifestations of RA

It is not possible to compare the occurrence of articular features and extra-articular manifestations described in section 2.2.2 with the figures for other countries. A good deal of the information contained in section 2.2.2 is based on data from abroad, and where both Dutch and foreign data are available, the differences in study methods rule out a satisfactory comparison.

2.3.3 Quality of life of RA-patients

To date no studies have been carried out which compare the quality of life of RA-patients in different countries. Such a comparison would be made extremely difficult by the current lack of standardization and international sociocultural differences. A project was, however, recently started (Euridiss), in which nine European countries are taking part and in which the influence of the health care system and the informal care system (social network) on the course of the disease and the quality of life of persons with a chronic disease is being studied. Currently RA is the subject of study (202). Despite this, it is not possible to make any statements regarding the quality of life of Dutch RA-patients in comparison with RA-patients in other countries. Quality-of-life studies have been carried out in some other countries, however, and it is likely that the findings also apply to the Dutch situation. A number of topics which have been studied abroad and which are also important for Dutch RA-patients are discussed below.

As discussed earlier in section 2.2.2.2, *pain* is one of the greatest drawbacks of RA for many patients. The pain arises not only as a result of the inflammation in the joints, but can also be a component of the systemic pathological process or can arise as a result of changes in pain thresholds. Side-effects of drugs can also produce pain (e.g. stomach pain after taking NSAIDs). A study of 729 rheumatology patients, of whom 60% were suffering from RA, showed that the medical consumption of patients with pain is greater, and the general health poorer, than that of patients with less pain. In patients with physical and psychological restrictions, this difference was much less clear-cut, in addition to which the level of pain was related to the physical restrictions. Other researchers also found that, particularly during active periods of the disease, the pain largely determines the level of physical restriction and the general level of health (123, 203, 204).

A study of hospitalized RA-patients showed that they scored higher on a *depression* scale than a control group of hospital patients and healthy people (120). A moderately higher score was also found among non-hospital patients (205). However, patients with other chronic diseases achieved scores of roughly the same level (120). On the basis of certain criteria (DSM III), 26% of RA-patients treated in outpatient clinics suffer from slight, chronic depression, while 17% suffer from severe depression (134). Longitudinal studies have shown that RA-patients with a higher level of depression are more frequently restricted in their daily activities after some years than those who are less depressive (123).

It should be noted here that a high score on the depression scale may also be an indication of physical symptoms of the disease. For example, tiredness can be a symptom both of RA and of depression. However, Zaphiroporelos and Burry, using a method designed to limit this difficulty as far as possible, found some form of depression in 46% of hospitalized RA-patients, compared with 19% of the control group (206).

Several researchers have found that the feelings of *helplessness* experienced by RA-patients are related to depression, reduced self-respect, poor psychosocial adjustment, deteriorated socio-economic environment and restrictions in carrying out daily activities. No relationship with the duration of the disease has been found (140, 207).

Clinical reports suggest that RA also leads to increased *anxiety*, though few indications of this are found in scientific studies. However, studies from 1971 did show that RA-patients scored higher in a questionnaire on emotions, anxiety, worries and tensions than healthy respondents (120).

Studies into the psychosocial adjustment of RA-patients have shown that their *self-respect* is lower (208, 209), as is their level of *job satisfaction*; their level of *indifference*, by contrast, was higher than that of members of a healthy control group (209).

Studies carried out abroad show that a chronic disease such as RA has a great impact on the *family life* of the patient. Approximately 60% of patients state that a change has taken place in at least one aspect of their psychosocial functioning as a result of changes in their family life (120). A study of 158 RA-patients receiving outpatient treatment at a teaching hospital looked at their *social relationships*. A distinction was made between more and less close relationships. The findings showed that patients with a higher level of disease activity or more restrictions did not have fewer close relationships or a lower level of satisfaction with their close relationships than patients with lower levels of disease activity or healthy persons. RA-patients with restrictions did, however, have difficulty in maintaining contacts with friends and acquaintances; this applied particularly to patients from a low socio-economic background. Both close and less close relationships had an influence on psychological well-being, although the link was stronger as regards the existence of and satisfaction with less close relationships (210). The need felt for personal relationships may well motivate patients to maintain a certain level of functioning. It can be observed that patients who are able to continue to maintain their personal relationships are ultimately less restricted in their daily functioning (123, 211).

An American study monitored 75 RA-patients between 1973 and 1982. The group consisted of 22 men and 53 women, whose average age in 1973 was 55 and who at that time had suffered from the disease for an average of 11 years. Of those who were still in full-time *employment* at the onset of the disease and who were below the age of 65 in 1973, only 40% were still employed in 1973. Only 36% of those who were younger than 65 in 1982 and who were still employed in 1973 were still working in 1982, and only 15% of those who were working at the onset of the disease (127).

A separate study looked at 245 RA-patients between the ages of 21 and 65 (both hospital patients and outpatients), who had suffered from the disease for an average of 9 years. 59% of the patients who were employed at the onset of the disease were no longer in a full-time job. In more than 80% of the cases this was attributable to RA. Important predictive variables for loss of employment were workplace conditions (flexibility) and duration and severity of the disease. There was no difference on the basis of socio-demographic category. Persons who were employed at the onset of the disease had since lost an average of 50% of their *earnings* (212).

Yelin found that the probability of *incapacity for work* was 33% for patients in whom the RA had been diagnosed less than five years previously. For patients who were known to have had the disease for longer than five years and who were in a more serious stage of the disease, the probability was as high as 70%. Yelin also found that persons who were more or less able to determine their own working pace as well as the type of activities and the hours worked per day, became incapacitated for work less quickly (213).

An American study of 5,652 persons from the open population showed that 56% of males with RA and 31% of females with RA were employed; this compared with figures for persons with no rheumatic disease of 89% and 62%, respectively. The *earnings* of men and women with RA were 48% and 27%, respectively, of the earnings of people without rheumatic disease. Approximately one third of this earnings loss was explained by the arthritis. Other explanations included more advanced age, lower level of education and multiple pathology (214).

On the basis of this survey of foreign research, it can be concluded that:

- Pain is largely responsible for the general state of health and medical consumption by RA-patients;
- RA-patients exhibit more symptoms of depression than healthy persons;
- RA has negative consequences for family life;
- RA appears to have little impact on the number of or satisfaction with close social relationships. The maintaining of these relationships demands a good deal of effort from patients with restrictions, particularly if they come from a lower socio-economic background;
- A large proportion of RA-patients become incapacitated for work as a result of the disease. Persons who are able more or less to determine the intensity and duration of the work themselves generally become incapacitated for work less quickly;
- The earnings of RA-patients are often greatly reduced after the onset of the disease.

2.3.4 Medical consumption as a result of RA

No international comparative studies have been carried out on medical consumption as a result of RA. Data for the various countries are, however, available regarding the uptake of care in general as a result of rheumatoid arthritis. A great deal of caution is necessary, however, when comparing Dutch figures for medical consumption with data from abroad: medical consumption results from a range of factors such as the prevalence of the disease, severity of the disease, medical therapeutic strategy, level of facilities available, funding system, etc. All these factors can vary from country to country, and it is often not clear which factors are responsible for an observed difference. In addition, the figures for medical consumption are partly determined by the method and accuracy of data collection and analysis and the diagnostic criteria adopted. In the light of these factors, it was decided not to draw any comparisons between the uptake figures found for the Netherlands and data from abroad.

2.4 Past trends and backgrounds to these trends

2.4.1 Occurrence of RA

No reliable data are available on the occurrence of RA. All the available data are inadequate and are subject to considerable distortion (bias). In order to make reliable statements about trends in RA, a large population (at least 500,000) needs to be monitored over many years (215) in accordance with standardized methods.

On the other hand, it is striking that the available data are relatively consistent in showing a reduction in the incidence of RA in recent decades, particularly among women (27, 216, 217, 218, 219). The latter may be due to the use of the oral contraceptive pill (220). There are also indications that RA is becoming a less severe disease (217), though recent findings suggest that the pill may be preventing the disease from becoming progressively more severe (53). It is highly possible that the fall in incidence is only an apparent one, due to the fact that it was more difficult in the past to distinguish RA-related diseases from RA itself.
It can be **concluded** that no clear statements can be made at the moment regarding possible falling trends in the incidence and severity of RA. Monitoring of a large population may offer more insight (blank spot).

2.4.2 Articular features and extra-articular manifestations of RA

As explained in section 2.2.2, reliable epidemiological figures on the occurrence of articular features and extra-articular manifestations of RA are scarce. As a result, it is difficult to indicate trends for the majority of these features and manifestations. There are, however, indications that severe generalized vasculitis is a relatively rare occurrence nowadays (81). Amyloidosis was formerly diagnosed among approximately 20% of patients with a disabling form of arthritis, whereas today it is rarely diagnosed (83). The incidence of infections among RA-patients has probably increased as a result of the increasing use of corticosteroids and immunosuppressives (93).

2.4.3 Quality of life of RA-patients

Major developments have taken place in the medical treatment of RA, which have an impact on the quality of life. The most obvious consequences of this have to do with physical well-being, though these developments have undoubtedly also had an impact on psychosocial well-being.

Improvements in both medical and surgical therapy mean that only a few patients now become so severely disabled that they are eventually forced to take to bed and/or wheelchair. New treatment methods in the area of physiotherapy have also played a part here. It is therefore highly likely that, in general, the physical well-being of RA-patients has improved substantially over recent decades. On the other hand, the new treatment patterns involve the use of more aggressive medication at an earlier stage in the disease, and possibly to the more frequent occurrence of side-effects. Reliable quantitative data on these developments are unfortunately not (yet) available.

Little is also known about possible developments in psychological and social well-being, though virtually all care-providers now acknowledge that RA can be accompanied by major psychosocial problems. A number of general social developments, such as individualization and the formation of smaller family units, will undoubtedly have had an effect on the social well-being of RA-patients, for example in the form of reduced social support.

Increasing emphasis has been placed on providing patients with information. In recent years education programmes have actually been developed specially for RA-patients, with the aim among other things of stimulating self-care by the patient. In the area of district nursing, too, an ever-increasing emphasis is now being placed on self-reliance.

Another positive development is that more account is now (rightly) being taken of the need for access by the less able-bodied in the design of public buildings. Housing corporations also appear to be devoting more attention to constructing modifiable dwellings, something which until recently received scant attention. In addition, existing buildings are also regularly modified.

In spite of the advances, however, there have also been some setbacks in recent years. Patients feel that some things have deteriorated, and there is anxiety for the future. These worries mainly relate to the patient's own financial contribution, cutbacks in physiotherapy, the slow improvement in - and in a number of cases actually decreasing - opportunities for participation in paid employment (despite the Handicapped Employees (Employment) Act), and the cutbacks in invalidity benefits.

2.4.4 Medical consumption as a result of RA

Lack of information makes it impossible to plot trends in medical consumption as a result of rheumatoid arthritis very far back in time. There follows a brief discussion of general trends in medical consumption, followed by a description of recent developments in the care structure and care-provision for RA and trends in uptake of care facilities as a result of rheumatoid arthritis.

A major problem in describing trends in the uptake of care is the changes in the composition and size of the relevant patient group as a result of demographic shifts. Other factors also make the description of trends difficult, such as possible autonomous developments in the disease incidence, changes in diagnostic criteria, etc. The literature on this subject usually does not correct for these potentially distorting variables, sometimes due to lack of data.

General developments in medical consumption

Although the medical consumption is largely determined by the occurrence of a disease and its duration and severity (objectively determined morbidity), social changes and developments on the supply side of the care system have had a particular influence on changes in the uptake of care.

The importance of the care provided by the informal care network has declined sharply in recent decades. This is the result both of social developments which have led to weaker social bonds (e.g. secularization, increased mobility, smaller families in which the grandparents do not live in, individualization), and also of the trend towards professionalization and "medicalization" (for example as a result of the increased possibilities of medicine, increased patient assertiveness and a changed attitude towards professional medical consumption). In view of the complementary nature of the relationship between informal and professional care, this has led to increased demand on professional medical care. In recent years, however, emphasis has been placed - particularly by the government - on substitution of care. This entails a shift from professional to informal care, and from secondary care to care in the domestic situation. Doubts have been voiced from various sides, however, as to the feasibility of this policy.

Reliable quantitative consumption data, which could be used to support the developments described above, are not available for a longer period. One possible indicator is the share taken by health care in the gross national product. During the period 1972-1982 this share rose from 6.8% to 8.6%, and subsequently continued to fluctuate around the 1982 level (2.2.1).

As regards the extent and composition of the medical consumption, data are available illustrating the trends over the last ten years. Data from the CBS Health Interview Survey covering the period 1981-1988 (2.2.2) indicate that the number of people consulting a general practitioner in the course of a single year increased slightly from 69.3% to 72.4%. The number of contacts per person in the population in the same period showed no change. During the same period the percentage of people consulting a specialist in the course of a single year and the average number of contacts per person per year remained stable. The same is true of the percentage of people admitted to hospital and the average number of admissions. There was, however, a steady fall in the length of stay in hospital during the period 1978-1988 (189). If only those people aged 65 and above are considered, an increase can be observed in the frequency of hospital admission during the period 1981-1985. This may be due to the increased treatment possibilities as a result of technological developments (2.2.3).

It can be concluded that the decline in the importance of the informal network and the trend towards "medicalization" and professionalization have led in the past to an increase in the uptake of care. Current government policy is geared to substitution of care, with a shift from secondary/-tertiary health care to primary/"pre-primary" health care. Although no extensive information on trends is available it can be tentatively concluded that the role of the general practitioner and the specialist have remained virtually unchanged over recent decades. Two striking features are the general fall in average length of stay in hospital and the increase in admission frequency among older people.

Trends in medical consumption as a result of RA
In addition to the general trends in medical consumption outlined above, a number of specific developments have taken place with respect to RA-care. Recent developments in this area include the following:

- Improved medication;
- Improved surgery;
- Small-scale deployment of rheumatology nurses (or hospital and community-based nurses) at rheumatology clinics;
- Experiments with ergotherapy in primary health care;
- The setting up of (re)training courses for general practitioners and physiotherapists.

It is not possible at this moment in time to assess what the consequences of these developments have been on the extent and composition of the medical consumption, since the majority of these developments are only recent, and their coverage is therefore generally still rather low.

Reliable (though non-standardized) data on Dutch trends in medical consumption as a result of rheumatoid arthritis are in fact only available for hospital and nursing home care. The number of hospital admissions as a result of rheumatoid arthritis (excluding juvenile RA) increased during the period 1980-1989 by 17%. The average length of stay per admission declined by almost 50% in the same period (from 43 days in 1980 to 24 days in 1989) (189). In nursing homes, the share of rheumatoid arthritis as one of the first three admission diagnoses in the total number of admissions remained reasonably stable during the period 1984-1989 (195).

2.5 Future developments

Reviewing the developments to date, it is evident that, broadly speaking, the epidemiology of RA is governed by three major background factors: demography, risk factors and medical technology (with respect to therapy). The diagrammatic representation of the epidemiology of RA as presented in Figure 2.1 can be extended with the aid of these background factors. Figure 2.5 illustrates the direct influence of these factors.

Figure 2.5 Background factors of importance for the epidemiology of RA

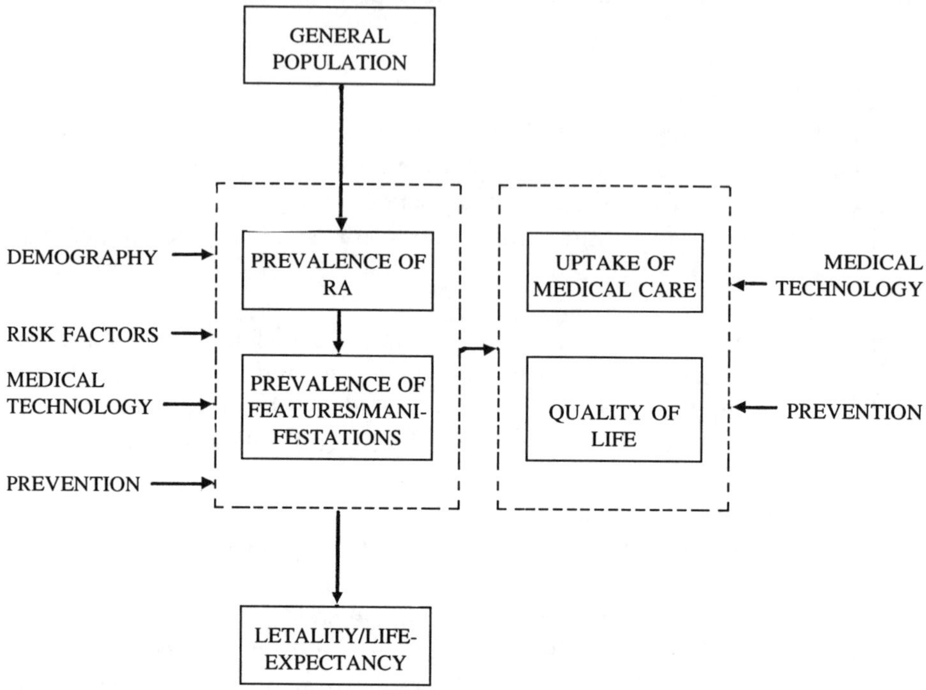

Clearly, future developments will also be determined by these same factors. Possible future developments in these fields are discussed briefly in section 2.5.1. Section 2.5.2 examines the potential for influencing future developments in RA, with particular attention being focused on preventive measures.

2.5.1 Significant background factors

Demography

As discussed in section 2.2.1, the incidence and prevalence of RA are dependent on age and sex. This means that demographic changes have an influence on the occurrence of RA. Population forecasts up to the year 2005 indicate an ageing of the population. It will be clear that an ageing of the Dutch population will result in an increase in the number of patients with RA, since prevalence increases with age. Given this increase in the number of patients with RA, it is highly likely that demographic changes will be accompanied by an absolute increase in the number of articular features and extra-articular manifestations of RA.

Risk factors
Greater insight has been gained in recent decades into the abnormal reaction of the immune system, possibly due to the effects of primary causal agents in immunogenetically predisposed persons. Modulation of the immune system is likely to become an important tool in the near future in tackling the problem of RA. A good deal remains unclear about immunogenetic predisposition and this applies even more so to the primary causal agents.

Medical technology
Past developments in medical technology which have had the most visible impact on the clinical picture of RA lie in the area of therapy. On the one hand there have been advances in medical treatment. Apart from the fact that new medicines for treating RA have been introduced which effect the immune system (including azathioprine and methotrexate), changes have also taken place in the treatment strategy. At the moment there is a clear trend away from a regime involving a staged progression to ever more powerful drugs, towards a strategy in which these powerful drugs are used at an early stage of the disease. On the other hand, there has been a good deal of progress in rheumatological surgery, particularly as regards prosthetic implantation. In addition to hip and knee prostheses, prostheses for other joints are being implanted or developed. Shoulder replacements are already a regular occurrence, while ankle prostheses are beginning to show promise and elbow prostheses are under development.

2.5.2 Scope for intervention

The cope for intervention includes measures in the field of prevention, where a distinction should be drawn between primary, secondary and tertiary prevention. *Primary prevention* is designed to prevent the onset of RA, while *secondary prevention* focuses on achieving the earliest possible intervention in the disease process in order to prevent permanent joint damage (Van Rijswijk, Groningen, personal communication). *Tertiary prevention* is designed to prevent the disease from becoming a chronic disorder which ultimately leads to permanent invalidity.

In the context of **primary prevention** it is important to be aware that both a genetic disposition and exposure to primary causal agents are important for the onset of RA. Influencing the genetic predisposition would only be possible through genetic manipulation, and it is possible to do no more than speculate on potential primary causal agents. It will be clear from this that primary prevention for RA is currently not a realistic possibility.

Within the context of rheumatology, **secondary prevention** can be defined as the detection of a disease at a stage in which *no (significant) joint damage* is yet present. Given the increased understanding of immunological disorders which has been gained in recent years, there may be possibilities for halting the progress of the disease by influencing the immune system (immune therapy), enabling permanent joint damage to be prevented or limited. For adequate secondary prevention it is absolutely essential that patients with RA are diagnosed as such at an early stage, so that early treatment can follow (47). In the majority of patients with RA substantial joint damage, which can be observed using X-Rays, occurs within the first two years of the onset of the disease. Once it has occurred, joint damage is probably irreversible and a damaged joint is subject to greatly accelerated wear (secondary arthrosis).

At the moment, however, there are no adequate diagnostic techniques, such as unique biological markers, which enable RA to be detected with certainty at an early stage of the disease. Available markers (including HLA DR-4, rheumatoid factor) are also frequently found among the general population, while they can be absent in patients with RA. There could be an important role here for the general practitioner, who is generally the first person to be confronted with the patient's complaints.

Tertiary prevention plays an extremely important role in RA. A number of aspects can be distinguished here. In the first place, depending on the complaints, an adequate medical therapy should be initiated (see Appendix 1). It is not possible to give general guidelines here, since the therapy needs to be matched to the complaints pattern and the personal circumstances of the patient. It is essential that the treating physician (rheumatologist) regularly monitors the patient.

Subsequently, (advice on) dosed rest, physiotherapy (particularly exercise therapy) and the use appliances and adaptation of the surroundings (ergotherapy) should be considered essential elements of the therapy. The psychosocial aspects should not be neglected here, and keeping patients informed is an extremely important part of this.

A last, extremely important element of tertiary prevention is surgery. The implantation of artificial joints can be described as the most spectacular contribution here. Improvements in the quality of prostheses and surgical techniques, which mean that the prostheses last longer, have made it possible to operate on younger patients as well as older ones.

It is highly likely that the various forms of tertiary prevention have a positive impact on the severity of the disease with its articular features and extra-articular manifestations, and on the quality of life. The effect on medical consumption, however, is more difficult to assess. If those RA-patients who are not yet known are diagnosed more frequently in the future, medical consumption will initially rise (irrespective of demographic changes). It is not unlikely, however, that early recognition of RA-patients followed by adequate treatment will in the long term result in a fall in medical consumption as a result of RA.

3 DELPHI STUDY OF POSSIBLE FUTURE DEVELOPMENTS. Results of an opinion survey among 30 experts

3.1 Outline of method used

3.1.1 Experts' forecasts

Once the current situation has been outlined, a scenario study proceeds to generate ideas on possible future developments. Various lines of approach can be used, and in the scenario study on RA the forecasts of experts were collected, a method also used in the scenario studies on diabetes mellitus and CNSLD and in several other scenario studies. This particular line of approach was the most appropriate for this research project, since the formulation of expectations about the future involves a subjective judgement. While the opinion of experts may include a degree of speculation, it is nevertheless more valuable than that of non-experts or interested laymen. Moreover, questioning experts from a range of backgrounds and disciplines made it possible to cover all aspects of RA in adequate detail.

3.1.2 Delphi method: workshop

Research into experts' forecasts can be approached in several different ways: the most important are sometimes called "subjective iterative group processes". This term implies that a group of experts is given the opportunity to express opinions on a particular subject in a situation of mutual interaction (this also allows for the adjustment of personal attitudes). The "brainstorm method" and the more formalized, written Delphi method both belong to this family of techniques. The latter method was used for this study, as a number of the questions required clear and precise answers. Written questionnaires are a more efficient method for this purpose than group discussions.

The Delphi method can be used to assemble the building blocks for compiling future scenarios, though a drawback of this method is that the interrelationships between forecasts cannot be shown clearly. These interrelationships are of major importance for the construction of scenarios, for example to ensure internal consistency. In order to amalgamate the scenario building blocks on a sound basis, a workshop was organized to round off the Delphi study. A number of the experts on the panel, as well as members of the Scenario Committee and the research team, took part in this workshop. A concluding meeting such as this also provides an opportunity to evaluate the plausibility of the research data and to examine methodological problems.

3.1.3 Practical elaboration

A panel of 35 experts was put together for the Delphi study. One of the main criteria here was to achieve a balanced distribution of expertise in the specific subjects covered by the questionnaire. The experts were chosen in such a way that the panel consisted not only of members of the medical and paramedical professions but also of representatives of the most important organizations and groups in society, such as research institutes, industry, patient associations, government, health insurance funds and private health organizations. Although the members of the Chronic Diseases Scenario Committee were closely involved in the preparations for the Delphi study, they were not included in the group of invited experts.

The questionnaires were arranged in two rounds. After processing the first round, the results were returned to the respondents in order to allow them to adjust and/or elaborate on their answers. The response rate was a highly satisfactory 91% (counting only those who participated fully in both rounds).

Table 3.1 gives a summary of the number of invited and participating members of the panel.

As stated in section 2.5, it may be assumed that future developments with regard to the number of patients, the incidence and severity of articular features and extra-articular manifestations of the disease, quality of life, life expectancy, medical consumption and the level of self-care will be determined by "autonomous background developments" (i.e. demography, changes in the risk factors and medico-technological developments) on the one hand and "policy interventions" on the other. This principle was central in the questionnaire design.

Table 3.1 Invited and participating members of the panel

	Invited	Participation round 1	round 2
Basic health care			
- socio-medical	1	1	0
Primary health care			
- general practitioners	3	3	3
- area nurses	2	2	2
- ergotherapists	1	1	1
Secondary and tertiary health care			
- rheumatologists	9	7	7
- orthopaedic surgeons	2	2	2
- hand plastic surgeon	1	1	1
- rehabilitation physician	1	1	1
- rheumatology nurses	2	2	2
- ergotherapists	2	2	2
- physiotherapists	1	1	1
- social work/psychologists	1	1	1
Research			
- behavioural science	1	1	1
- epidemiological	1	1	1
- pharmaceutical	2	2	2
- economic	1	1	1
Social groupings			
- patient associations	1	1	1
- National Rheumatism Fund	1	1	1
- government	1	1	1
- Health Insurance Fund Council	1	1	1
- Association of Dutch Health Insurers	1	1	1
Total	35	33	32

The questionnaire sought to elicit the experts' forecasts regarding the development of RA up to the year 2005 with regard to the following variables:

- incidence (the number of new patients);
- incidence and severity of articular features;
- incidence and severity of extra-articular manifestations;
- quality of life;
- life expectancy;
- demand for care and medical consumption;

In the first round the experts were asked which future developments they though most likely. They were then asked to indicate what developments or measures they considered should be stimulated by the government or other social groups in order to reach the year 2005 in the most advantageous circumstances.

The main aim of the second round was to confront the respondents with the answers obtained from the rest of the panel in relation to their own answers. Another important aim was to provide feedback on the internal inconsistencies between individual forecasts as indicated in the answers, and to request adjusted answers. A number of issues, including underdiagnosis, life expectancy and in-hospital rheumatology care, were dealt with in more detail. The respondents were asked to *leave out of consideration* the impact of *demographic developments* such as ageing, since this could be calculated separately from existing data (cf. section 4.2.2).

One drawback in carrying out an exclusively written survey is that interrelationships between expectations cannot be expressed clearly. In addition, since the expected developments appeared to contain a number of inconsistencies which demanded discussion, a workshop was organized in which the results of the Delphi study were presented and a number of provisional scenarios were discussed in more detail. The measures which had been formulated in general terms in the responses to the questionnaire were also defined more specifically. A selection of the respondents from the Delphi study took part in this workshop, along with the RA-experts from the Scenario Committee and the members of the research team. In the selection of these panel members, too, an attempt was made to achieve a proportional distribution across the various medical and paramedical professions and social groupings.

Information was presented during the workshop which could be used in the interpretation of the responses given by the participants in the Delphi study and in the construction of the definitive scenarios. In a few cases the expectations of the Delphi panel were adjusted. The results of the workshop were integrated as far as possible into the description of the results of the Delphi study. Where the participants in the workshop expressed different expectations from those of the Delphi panel, this is clearly indicated.

Table 3.2 shows the type of questions used in the Delphi study, enabling the reader to form an impression of the content of the questionnaires.

Table 3.2 Examples of questions used in the Delphi study on RA

---

1. The number of persons in the Dutch population (per 10,000) with a genetic predisposition to developing RA in the period 1990-2005
   0 is increasing
   0 shows no change
   0 is decreasing
   0 is unknown

2. Do you suspect that, apart from bacteria and viruses, there are also *other* important exogenous factors which have a causal link with RA?

3. Do you expect any changes in the period 1990-2005 in the degree of exposure to the exogenous factors you have named in answer to question 2 (including bacteria and viruses)?
   To which of these factors do you expect exposure to increase in the period 1990-2005?
   To which do you expect exposure to decrease?

4. To what extent do you expect the incidence of RA in the year 2005 to have changed with respect to the year 1990?
   0 increase of ...%
   0 no change
   0 decrease of ...%

The respondents were consistently asked to explain why they expected particular developments.

Since the questionnaire covered a wide range of disciplines and fields, the participants were not expected to consider themselves experts in all areas. The panel members were therefore asked at the end of the first questionnaire to indicate their level of expertise in each subject. The analysis includes only those respondents who considered themselves sufficiently qualified.

On average approximately 22% of the respondents for each section considered themselves *non*-expert. Of the remaining 78% approximately half considered themselves fully qualified and half partly qualified in that particular subject. A strikingly high number of respondents considered themselves qualified on the quality of life, provision of and demand for care and medical consumption. By contrast, only a small number considered themselves expert on fundamental research, diagnosis and medication therapy.

3.2 Results of the Delphi study

3.2.1 Introduction

The most important results of the Delphi study, including the workshop, are discussed below, with the main focus being on the principal forecasts of the panel. The size and composition (i.e. age and sex breakdown) of the population have been assumed to be static for the period 1990-2005, since the effect of demographic change is best calculated on the basis of mathematical models.

The discussion of most of the results is based on the respondents' answers to the questionnaire from the second Delphi round, supplemented by explanations obtained during the workshop. For each topic, a description is given only of the answers from those respondents who consider themselves (partially) qualified in that field. Some of the answers are set out in tables; in these cases the value "N" represents the number of experts on whom the table is based.

The first section (3.2.2) shows the estimates of expected developments with regard to the incidence, diagnosis, articular features, extra-articular manifestations, iatrogenic complications, physical function, quality of life, life expectancy, demand for care and medical consumption. Section 2.3.3 considers the grounds for these developments as put forward by the participants, followed in section 2.3.4 by the measures required to guide the developments along the most favourable lines. It should be stressed that the explanations of trends as described in this sector are those of the Delphi panel, and do not necessarily represent the views of the Chronic Diseases Scenario Committee.

It was not possible to reach consensus on every subject dealt with in the Delphi study. Where several opinions were extant, these have all been described, including minority standpoints - though these minority views did have to be supported by argument.

For the majority of topics, the views *within* certain disciplines varied just as much or as little as the views *between* the various disciplines. Where there are clear differences of opinion between disciplines, this is stated in the text.

3.2.2 Expected developments in the period 1990-2005

The most important results of the forecasts of the Delphi panel are summarized in Tables 3.3 and 3.4. The group responses in these tables relate to the opinions of more than *two-thirds* of the "experts".

Table 3.3 looks first at changes in incidence and rate of diagnosis, and second at changes *per RA-patient* in the severity of articular features, extra-articular manifestations, iatrogenic complications, physical function, quality of life and life expectancy. In Table 3.4 the assumption has been made in the questions that the incidence of RA and the rate of diagnosis remain unchanged. The first column shows the percentage of RA-patients under the care or treatment of a particular care facility. The second column shows the amount of care required per day by an "average" RA-patient who is under the care of a particular care facility.

Table 3.3 Summary of the main results of the Delphi study: developments up to the year 2005 with an unchanged demographic situation (N = 17-30)

Variable	Change		
Incidence (age-specific)		0	
Rate of diagnosis		+	
Articular features	Incidence:		Severity:
pain	0/-		0/-
functional impairment	0/-		-
deformity	0/-		-
Extra-art. manifestations	Incidence:		Severity:
tiredness	0		0/-
neurological disorders	0		0
Sjögren's syndrome	0		0
vasculitis	0		0
Felty's syndrome	0		0
amyloidosis	0/-		0/-
renal impairment*	0		0
septic arthritis	0		0
Iatrogenic complications	+/0		0
Physical function		+	
Quality of life		+/0	
Life expectancy		+/0	

* Not as a result of amyloidosis

Key to codes:
++ = strong increase
\+ = moderate increase
0 = no change
\- = moderate decrease
-- = strong decrease

Table 3.4 Summary of the main results of the Delphi study with regard to expected demand for care: developments up to the year 2005 with unchanged demographic situation, incidence and rate of diagnosis (N = 31)

	Percentage RA-patients receiving care	Daily demand for care per patient receiving care
Primary health care		
general practitioners	+/0	+/0
district nursing	+/0	+/0
physiotherapy	+/0	+/0
ergotherapy	+	+
home help	+	+
Secondary health care		
outpatient clinic	+	+
clinic	0/-	+/0 *
Tertiary health care		
specialized rheumatology hospital	+/0/-	+/0/- *
nursing home	0/-	+/0 *
rest home	0	+/0

* Adjusted following the workshop

Key to codes:
+ = moderate increase
0 = no change
- = moderate decrease

The results of these tables are discussed in more detail below.

Incidence of rheumatoid arthritis

According to 81% of the respondents (N = 15) there will be no change in the incidence of RA in the period 1990-2005. 10% expect an increase in incidence and 5% a decrease. The median of the expected changes is an increase of 0% (the median is the mid-value when responses are arranged in order of size). The minimum and maximum values stated were -10% and +5%, respectively.

Underdiagnosis

The panel was asked to answer the questions on changes in the incidence on RA independently of any increase or decrease in the interest shown by (para)medical personnel (in particular general practitioners) and/or society in RA. If this changed interest were taken into account, this would lead to an increase or decrease in the number of RA-patients diagnosed as such.

With one exception, all respondents (N = 20) expect to see an increase over the coming 15 years in the percentage of RA-patients who are actually diagnosed as suffering from the disease. The panel estimates that at the present approximately 50% of RA-patients are *known* to be sufferers by their physician (who may be their GP). The panel expects this percentage to increase to 60% over the next 15 years. The spread of these percentages was fairly wide.

These estimates are based on the assumption that diagnostic techniques will not change in this period. However, 59% of the respondents (N = 17) feel that major changes will take place in this area which could lead equally well to more frequent or less frequent diagnosis of RA. The reason for a potential decrease in diagnosis is that better diagnostic techniques could mean that in a number of cases the disease proves not to be RA but a different disorder. According to 47% of respondents, the net result of diagnostic changes will be an increase in the number of RA-patients detected each year. A further 47% expect no change in this respect, and only 6% expect to see a decrease in this number.

Possible therapeutic developments

Overall, 88% of the respondents expect to see an improvement in the therapeutic facilities available to RA-patients. The remainder expect no significant changes. No-one expects a deterioration in the facilities (N = 25).

Articular features of RA

The panel was asked to indicate the expected changes in the incidence and severity of articular features. Table 3.5 sets out these expectations. The figures relate to the percentage of respondents in each case. If the sum of the percentages of respondents is less than 100%, this is because a number of respondents did not answer a particular question.

The percentage of patients who will experience pain, functional impairment or deformities will remain unchanged or decrease according to the panel, as will the severity of these articular features.

Table 3.5 Expected changes in incidence and severity of three major articular features of RA in the period 1990-2005 (N=27)

Feature of RA		+	0	-	Total
Pain:	incidence	4	56	41	0/-
	severity	4	44	52	0/-
Functional impairment:	incidence	0	41	59	0/-
	severity	0	37	63	-
Deformity:	incidence	4	37	59	0/-
	severity	4	30	67	-

Key to codes:
+ = increase
0 = no change
- = decrease

Extra-articular manifestations

The panel was also asked to indicate what changes it expected in the incidence and severity of eight extra-articular manifestations of RA and iatrogenic complications. Table 3.6 shows these forecasts.

Most of the respondents expect both the incidence and the severity of the majority of extra-articular manifestations to remain more or less unchanged in the period 1990-2005. The only two exceptions are the incidence and severity of amyloidosis and tiredness, which a majority of the group expect to remain unchanged or fall. The participants in the workshop held the view that whether the incidence and severity of extra-articular manifestations - with the exception of amyloidosis - will change is still completely unknown. As regards the incidence of iatrogenic complications, a majority of the Delphi panel expect to see this increase or remain at the same level, although some general practitioners, rheumatologists, surgeons and researchers hold the opposite view and expect a fall.

Table 3.6 **Expectations regarding the change in incidence and severity of eight major extra-articular manifestations of RA and iatrogenic complications in the period 1990-2005 (N = 22-25).**

Complication		Percentage of respondents +	0	-	Total*
Tiredness:	incidence	0	70	26	0
	severity	0	59	37	0/-
Neurological disorders:	incidence	9	64	14	0
	severity	0	82	5	0
Sjögren's syndrome:	incidence	9	64	5	0
	severity	0	68	9	0
Vasculitis:	incidence	9	61	17	0
	severity	0	70	17	0
Felty's syndrome:	incidence	0	73	5	0
	severity	0	64	14	0
Renal impairment**:	incidence	18	46	18	0
	severity	5	59	18	0
Amyloidosis:	incidence	9	52	26	0/-
	severity	0	65	22	0/-
Septic arthritis:	incidence	9	65	13	0
	severity	4	74	9	0
Iatrogenic complications:	incidence	35	35	22	+/0
	severity	22	49	22	0

* Total: roughly speaking the group response represents the opinion of more than two-thirds of the "experts". For an explanation of codes see Table 3.5.

** Not as a result of amyloidosis.

Quality of care-provision
81% of the respondents (N = 31) expect the quality of care-provision, disregarding therapeutic changes, to improve. 16% forecast no change in this respect, and only 3% expect to see a deterioration.

Quality of life
53% of the respondents (N = 30) expect to see some improvement in the psychosocial component of the quality of life of RA-patients in the period 1990-2005. 3% expect to see a significant improvement, 33% expect no change and 7% expect to see a slight worsening of the psychosocial component.

Life expectancy
The questionnaires described a "typical" Dutch RA-patient (see Annex 6). Members of the panel were asked whether the life expectancy of a patient diagnosed in 2005 will have increased or decreased compared to a similar patient diagnosed in 1990. Panellists were asked to assume an unchanging life expectancy among the general population.

Of the 22 (partially) qualified respondents, 63% expect the life expectancy of the patient to have increased, 25% expect no change and 8% expect the life expectancy to have decreased. The median of the difference forecast by the respondents in life expectancy between a patient diagnosed in 2005 and a patient diagnosed in 1990 is +1 year (minimum and maximum = -1 and +6 years, respectively).

Demand for care and medical consumption
The respondents expect that, for an unchanged population of RA-patients, *the percentage of RA-patients* who are receiving primary health care or outpatient treatment will increase. The percentage of RA-patients under the care of clinics and nursing homes is expected to decrease somewhat while the percentage being cared for in rest homes is expected to remain more or less unchanged. There is a difference of opinion over the development in the percentage of patients under the care of specialized rheumatology hospitals (see Table 3.4).

The *amount* of care required *per day* by an *"average" RA-patient who is under the care* of the primary health care system, outpatient clinic, clinic, nursing home or rest home, will increase according to the panel. Such patients will make more frequent and greater demands on these forms of care.

3.2.3 Underlying causes of the expected changes

In order to understand the future developments it is important to describe the causes or mechanisms upon which the panel members have based their expectations. These subjects are discussed in this section. For the sake of clarity not all the results are mentioned. If, for example, a large majority of the respondents expects an increase, there would seem little point in including the answers of the respondents with a differing opinion. However, where there was little consensus about the expected developments, several arguments have been described here.

Incidence

A change in the incidence of RA could be explained by:

a. a relative increase or decrease in the occurrence of *genetic predisposition* to RA among the population.
b. an increase or decrease in the level of exposure of the population to (a) particular *exogenous factor(s)*.

Assuming the size and composition of the population remains static, no-one expects to see either an increase or a decrease in the period 1990-2005 in the number of persons with a genetic predisposition to developing RA per 10,000 inhabitants. 76% of the respondents expect the number to remain the same as there is no reason to expect changes in the distribution of the genetic material (HLA) among the population, and because the incidence of RA over the past 15 years has also undergone no change. The remaining 24% state that we do not know the answer because there is simply too little information available.

Apart from bacteria and viruses, 52% of the respondents consider that there are also *other* important exogenous factors which have a causal link with RA and which can (help to) activate a genetic predisposition for RA. The following factors were mentioned (figures between brackets are the percentage of respondents naming that factor):

- food and other allergens (29%)
- a wide range of aspecific factors (19%)
- chemical substances (environmental pollution) (14%)
- psychosocial factors (14%)
- emotional and physical stress (14%)
- overloading of joints (5%)

According to the respondents these are factors which could affect the immune system.

The remaining 48% of the respondents consider that there are no other exogenous factors which have a causal link with RA. The majority of the panel (67%) do *not* expect changes in the level of exposure to exogenous factors (including bacteria and viruses) which have a causal link with RA. 29% do expect changes in the form of an increase in exposure to allergens, chemical substances and environmental pollutants, increasing societal complexity and more emotional and physical stress. According to this group there will be a decrease in overloading of joints as a factor.

A few respondents, while expecting changes, feel that the effects of the various factors could work in different directions, effectively cancelling each other out with a resultant net effect on incidence of nil.

Underdiagnosis

The members of the panel expect that more RA-patients will be known to their physician in 2005 than is the case in 1990. Several reasons are given for this. 70% of the respondents estimate that greater *expertise of general practitioners, in particular* in the period 1990-2005 will lead to less serious RA-patients being referred to specialists at an earlier stage, so that the diagnosis of RA will be established earlier. 65% of the respondents predict an increase in *patient assertiveness*, as a result of which patients will state at an earlier stage their wish to be referred to a specialist. 30% of the panel feel that, partly as a result of media attention, there will be *greater awareness among the "public"* with respect to diseases and clinical pictures. People will develop increased attention for their own bodies and will no longer be so ready to accept disorders. In addition, 55% of the panel expect that *access to specialists* will increase and that the distribution of specialists throughout the country will improve.

Apart from these non-technical developments, 59% of the respondents (N = 15) also expect to see important developments in the diagnosis of RA. Factors mentioned include genetic research, immunological research, MRI (Magnetic Resonance Imaging) and serological testing. 71% of the respondents (N = 17) expect that such refined, improved and new diagnostic techniques will lead to earlier and more frequent diagnosis of RA. This could lead to a mixture of RA in the early stages, which is not progressing rapidly, and marginal diagnoses. New diagnostic criteria could also contribute to this: a number of patients who would not have been diagnosed as suffering from RA in 1990 would indeed be diagnosed as RA-patients in 2005 according to this view. On the other hand, 59% of the respondents (particularly rheumatologists) expect that improved diagnostic techniques and increased knowledge of cell and molecular biology (genetic mapping) will lead to the diagnosis of RA being split up into several diagnoses, with some people who would previously have been diagnosed as RA-patients being diagnosed as having a different disorder of the musculo-skeletal system. Such a development would then lead to the fall in the number of persons diagnosed as having RA.

Approximately half the panel feel that the net effect of these changes in diagnosis will be an increase in the number of RA-patients detected annually. The other half expect no change.

Possible therapeutic developments

Medication

The expected developments in medication are divided here into developments in existing medicines for treating RA, developments in medicines which are currently used for treating diseases other than RA, and new medicines.

There is broad consensus on the expected developments in *existing medications used for treating RA*. 87% of the respondents (N = 15) support the trends outlined below.

The greatest improvements are expected in NSAIDs (Non-Steroid Anti-Inflammatory Drugs). The expectation is that these will become less toxic, that they will be used more selectively, that the method of administering will improve, that preparations with a longer-lasting effect will appear on the market. A single respondent expressed doubt concerning the development of NSAIDs. The view was put forward during the workshop that little in the way of improvements can be expected from the present generation of NSAIDs; much more is expected of a subsequent generation, which will work according to a completely different mechanism.

Anti-malaria preparations, gold preparations and penicillamine may come to be used less in the future. According to the panel, their effects will not be improved to any significant extent. It is possible that sulphasalazine will be used more frequently, particularly in the early stage of the disease, and it will be combined more effectively with other treatments. The panel also expects that immunosuppressives will be used more frequently and administered at an earlier stage. Their toxicity will decrease and the emergence of a method of local administering is also possible. Developments are expected particularly in the area of immunomodulators.

Corticosteroids may be used more frequently, for bridging, since the panel feels that their toxicity will decrease. The expectation is that these drugs will be used more often in support of immunosuppressives.

Of all the *existing medicines* which are currently *used for treating diseases other than RA*, 55% of the 11 respondents predict that only cyclosporin (or other immunosuppressives) will be used to treat RA during the next 15 years, possibly being used in particular for serious RA-patients who are resistant to other medicines. As noted above, these substances are already in use to a limited extent for the treatment of RA.

Additionally, all respondents expect that *new medicines* will become available for the treatment of RA over the next 15 years. Examples given include the second generation of NSAIDs (55% of respondents); monoclonal antibodies targeted against cell receptors (55%) and against cytokins (harmful mediators) (27%); T-cell vaccination (45%); radical scavengers (27%); inhibitors of the enzymes collagenase, stromelysin and elastase, which probably play an important role in the breakdown of cartilage (27%); and omega-3 fatty acid precursors (9%).

According to the respondents, all the new medicines referred to would be used mainly for relatively serious patients who, as well as suffering from general malaise, are also subject to pain in the joints, slight to moderate swellings and morning stiffness. Only the new NSAIDs are expected to be used for RA-patients suffering only from general malaise (the division of RA into five stages as described by Harris has been used here (1)).

Surgery
All respondents (N = 17) expect improvements or innovations in surgery. Replacement prostheses, not only for the hip and knee joints, but also for the hand, shoulder, elbow and ankle for patients suffering from destructive changes and pain in these joints will improve according to 94% of the respondents. 88% forecast that these joint prostheses will also become useable for relatively young RA-patients. Similarly, 88% expect that less loosening and infections will arise. 82% consider that the quality of the joint implant material will improve, while 59% feel that the emphasis in operations of this type will shift towards surgery at an early stage in the disease process. 88% of respondents also expect that tendon reconstructions and repair of postural disorders, particularly of the hand, will improve. The techniques of synovectomies (the surgical removal of a damaged synovial membrane from the joint) are also expect to improve (65% of respondents).

Doubt is still expressed that cartilage transplants will be sufficiently developed to become an important factor in treatment, though 35% expect that this will be the case. Also important in this connection is the forecast that the multidisciplinary cooperation between the specialisms plastic surgery/hand surgery, rehabilitation and rheumatology will increase; this expectation was expressed by 76% of respondents.

Physiotherapy/exercise therapy
70% of the panel (N = 23) expect to see one or more improvements or innovations in physiotherapy and/or exercise therapy. 65% forecast that treatment programmes will begin earlier in the course of the disease. 61% expect that pain-control techniques will improve, and 61% expect that physiotherapy will be applied in a more aware and better way.

Structured exercise therapy will receive more attention and be more frequently available, especially early in the course of the disease (61% of respondents). 57% expect that fitness training will reduce tiredness.

49% of the panel expect that all of the above developments in the area of physiotherapy will occur. 30% expect no improvement at all.

74% of respondents feel that scientific research is necessary in order to assess the effectiveness of physiotherapy and if possible to improve its usefulness (through more specific application). Additionally, 65% of the respondents consider that the need for improvements in physiotherapy training with respect to RA should be examined.

Dietetics

According to 39% of the respondents (N = 13) it will not be possible through dietetics over the next 15 years to reduce the complaints of RA-patients for whom food allergies play a role in their symptomatology. However, the same percentage (39%) expect that some relief will be possible, and 23% expect that the symptomatology can be significantly reduced. According to them, it should be possible to influence the immune response by means of dietetics.

The number of RA-patients involved here is estimated by the respondents at 7.5% (minimum and maximum = 2% and 15%, respectively).

Alternative therapies

In the first round, 9% of the panel members indicated that they expected improvements or innovations in alternative therapies (N = 33). No distinction was made here between the various therapies.

43% of the panel were of the opinion that the effects of alternative therapies need to be studied further. 57% disagreed with this view (N = 21).

71% of the panel expect that a drastic reduction in the use of alternative therapies would be possible if the psychosocial support in rheumatology departments (as provided by social workers, psychologists, rheumatology consultants, etc.) were improved.

Articular features

The incidence and severity of the articular features of RA (pain, functional impairment and deformity) will reduce according to the panel. In their view, early establishment of the correct diagnosis and earlier administering of improved therapy will lead to postponement of such problems. The better (combinations of) treatment possibilities for RA lie in the areas of medication therapy, physiotherapy, surgery and rehabilitation. Important factors here are better information and instructions with regard to posture, load and movement. Finally, the panel feel that better possibilities will emerge for controlling pain and that patients, by learning pain control techniques, will be better able to cope with the pain.

Extra-articular manifestations and iatrogenic complications

The panel expects the incidence and severity of the majority of extra-articular manifestations to remain at approximately the same level. The participants in the workshop, however, felt that this was still an unknown factor; according to them, only the incidence and severity of *amyloidosis* will show a fall. An explanation for this is that the therapy used in treating RA concentrates in the first instance on reducing joint complaints and damage. Since the articular features of RA and amyloidosis have the same genesis, improvement in the diagnosis of RA and the treatment of joint problems (more aggressive therapies) will also lead to a reduction in incidence of amyloidosis. The other extra-articular manifestations, by contrast, have a different genesis. As a result, the workshop participants feel that therapeutic treatments have no effect here, or else the effect is still unknown. No reasons were given for the expected fall in the severity of *tiredness*. The incidence of *iatrogenic complications* could increase according to the panel for a number of reasons: new medicines will emerge with which little experience has been gained; new medicines will be more aggressive; secondary health care treatments will be employed in primary health care; and there will be increased potential for infections to occur during joint operations and arthroscopies, caused by resistant hospital bacteria.

Care provision

In the first round the members of the panel were asked to assess whether 35 possible developments would be important for the group of RA-patients in the next 15 years. In the case of 22 of these developments, more than 50% of the respondents felt that this would be the case. The panel also felt that most of these developments should receive additional stimulation (see section 3.2.4 "Care provision"). However, the panel also expected to see a number of developments which would not require additional stimulation, but which were expected to occur "autonomously". The most important of these are additional (in-service) training on RA for district and area nurses, treatment and diagnosis by rheumatologists according to protocols, improved training in rheumatology, additional (in-service) training of rheumatologists and intensification of the collaboration between different rheumatology centres and within the primary health care system.

Quality of life

Most respondents expect the psychosocial component of the quality of life of RA-patients to improve. This was explained on the basis of a number of developments which panel members expect to occur in the next 15 years. These are listed below in order of probability:

1. Increasing development and availability of appliances.
2. Increasing possibilities for RA-patients to carry out general daily activities.
3. Increasing patient assertiveness.
4. Increasing number of discussion groups/patient networks.
5. Increasing accessibility of buildings and public transport.
6. Increasing number of modifiable dwellings in urban centres.
7. Increasing disease awareness of patients.
8. Increasing public information about rheumatism.
9. Increasing self-care.
10. Decreasing dependence on others.
11. More frequent application of the Handicapped Employees (Employment) Act.
12. More frequent financial help for home adaptations and appliances.

In spite of these optimistic forecasts regarding the quality of life of RA-patients, the respondents were also aware of a number of developments and measures on the sociocultural plane which could have undesirable *adverse* effects. Again, these are listed below in order of probability:

1. Economic decline will lead to further cutbacks in health care, education and scientific research. Subsidies and financial schemes for modified facilities (housing), appliances and/or benefits will be cut back and the procedures for claiming them will become more complicated. Restrictive measures could be implemented with respect to the nature and scope of assistance, for example home help (leading among other things to overburdening of the informal care network), physiotherapy, medicines and psychosocial care.
2. The proposed structure and financing of health care in the Netherlands (e.g. the Dekker Plan and the Simons Plan) have adverse consequences. A basic package of health insurance or national insurance may be created which provides limited cover (excluding physiotherapy and medicines) and with a risk excess to be paid by the patient; this would increase the financial pressure on those suffering from chronic diseases (such as RA-patients), who are often less able to bear this pressure. As

a result, some patients will receive treatment too late, so that damage to joints will occur more frequently, leading in turn to the need for more expensive care (operations, intensive support).

3. More unemployment will arise among RA-patients. The Handicapped Employees (Employment) Act will be implemented inadequately and the qualifying age for early retirement will be increased. More emphasis on achievement and earnings in society will lead to a deterioration in the position of the RA-patient.
4. RA-patients will become lonely and socially isolated.
5. A colder society will mean less solidarity among the population. The sick and handicapped will suffer as a result of the generalization by politicians of all benefit-claimants.
6. RA-patients will not be involved in the design of the care which is targeted at them.

Life expectancy

Diverse reasons were given for the expected increase in life expectancy of RA-patients. These are listed below in order of priority. The first was cited by 54% of the respondents, the last by 25%:

1. Better prevention of extra-articular manifestations and iatrogenic complications, plus more rapid and better treatment of these problems.
2. better control of infection phenomena.
3. earlier diagnosis and treatment.
4. medical developments and increased attention for aspects of "care" will lead to an improvement in the welfare of patients and a decrease in psychosocial problems, which have an effect on life expectancy.
5. improvement in total care availability.

Reasons given for a possible unchanged life expectancy were as follows (also given in order of priority, and cited by between 25% and 8% of the respondents):

1. Better treatment (see above), while improving the quality of life, will have no effect on life expectancy.
2. While RA leads to death in only a minority of cases, it does reduce the quality of life.
3. The shortened life expectancy is based on *severe* extra-articular manifestations and iatrogenic complications. These will not decrease (particularly iatrogenic complications).

4. Knowledge of the risk factors and genetic factors which cause the shorter life expectancy will probably not increase greatly.
5. There will be no essential changes in the treatment.

Demand for care and medical consumption

General

Cutbacks will mean that substitution will be encouraged - substitution of professional care by informal care, of in-patient care by outpatient care, day-treatment and/or primary health care (home care). On the other hand, patients will demand more medical care in the future. While a proportion of these patients will go to their general practitioner, others will visit their GP less frequently and less readily, but will more frequently and more readily wish to consult a rheumatologist. This would then lead to more outpatient care. It should be emphasized once again that demographic developments have been left out of consideration in this section.

Care by general practitioners

As already stated, the increased emphasis on primary health care, and particularly home care, will result in a greater demand by chronic patients for care from their general practitioner. This will certainly be the case if the organization and content of primary health care improves.

Since professional training will focus more on rheumatic disease, and also as a result of additional (in-service) training, a large proportion of the panel expect the expertise of general practitioners with respect to RA to increase, making them better able to recognize RA and to detect RA-patients more actively. There was no consensus among the panel on the question of whether general practitioners will then refer these patients on or will treat them themselves.

District nursing care

Many respondents expect improved organization and content of primary health care to lead to a concomitant increase in the demand on the district nursing service. As a result, home nursing will become better coordinated and more flexible which in turn, apart from the substitution already referred to, will also lead to a shift from nursing home care to home care. As well as increasing the number of patients, this will also mean more serious patients, requiring more care. The emphasis will lie on enabling patients to function more or less independently in the domestic situation.

Increased cooperation with the secondary health care sector may also reinforce the substitution by primary health care. Although demand for informal care will increase, the amount of such care actually provided will decrease, and this will largely have to be accommodated by the district nursing service.

A few respondents wondered whether, in the light of economic cutbacks, the number of training places in the district nursing service will increase sufficiently.

Physiotherapy
Some respondents expect that improved organization and content of primary health care will also lead to an increase in the demand placed on physiotherapy. Here, too, the shift from nursing home care to home care will play a role.

More treatment methods will be available to physiotherapists. It will be possible to give patients more exercise instructions and the therapy will be initiated at an earlier stage in the course of the disease.

The majority of the panel expect the demand for physiotherapy to remain more or less unchanged. There may well be some changes in terms of content, however, such as better specialization and a greater concentration on home exercising.

A number of respondents commented that too much attention is currently being devoted to physiotherapy, which often proves to be ineffective. According to these panellists, it will be necessary to make better and more efficient use of physiotherapy, since otherwise other care-providers will take over the care.

Ergotherapy
The majority of the panel expect that ergotherapy will receive more attention in primary health care and will be employed more often, sometimes following a referral by the rheumatologist. Ergotherapy would fit in with the aim of making handicapped people more independent and would therefore improve the quality of life. There is some leeway to be made up in the area of ergotherapy.

Outpatient care
The panel was almost unanimous in expecting the demand for outpatient care to increase. Better diagnosis will enable general practitioners to detect more RA-patients, a proportion of whom will be referred to specialists, where specific treatment and guidance can be given. It is possible that more paramedical care will also be provided in outpatient clinics, for example by hospital and community-based nurses.

Hospital care
A large section of the panel considered that substitution to outpatient and home care will lead to a decrease in the percentage of RA-patients receiving hospital care. This substitution may then lead to an increase in the demand for care per admitted patient per day as a result of the concentration of seriously ill patients.

The increasing care in hospital rheumatology units, and the more targeted hospital treatment of RA, administered in accordance with protocols, is expected to lead to a fall in the hospitalization period of RA-patients.

Care in specialized rheumatology hospitals
The panel failed to produce a unanimous answer to the question as to whether there will be any reduction in the percentage of RA-patients in the care of specialized rheumatology hospitals. Those members of the panel who expect an increase in this percentage base this opinion on an expected increase in the level of expertise in these specialized hospitals (pooling of knowledge and development of a range of treatment methods), which in turn will create a greater demand for these services. If hospital admission becomes necessary, people will more frequently opt for this specialized care.

A number of respondents expect no change in the demand for care. According to this view a category of patients will remain for whom specialized rheumatology services continue to be necessary, and the size of this group will undergo little change. According to these respondents, the percentage of patients who will have to be put on medication, and the number of operations, will not change drastically.

In contrast to this view, several members of the panel expect that the care provided by specialized rheumatology hospitals will reduce, or even that these institutions will disappear.

Nursing home care
The panel expects demand for nursing home care (on the assumption of a static demographic situation) to remain at the same level or to decrease. The respondents do, however, expect an increase in day-treatment. As with rest home care (see below), the effect of an additional increase in the life expectancy of RA-patients has not been taken into account here. A possible decrease is expected to follow from the substitution of care and better treatment, as a result of which the capacities of patients will increase and, with the help of primary health care and support from the outpatient clinic, they will be able to remain in the domestic situation for longer. Concentration of seriously ill patients will lead to an increase of the demand for care per patient admitted.

Rest-home care
Most respondents expect the need for rest-home care to remain unchanged. On the one hand substitution of care may mean that a proportion of RA-patients will be able to manage with home care and ambulant care, while on the other hand, a proportion of the patients who would previously have gone to nursing homes will in future go to a rest home.

Since the number of patients requiring relatively less assistance will decrease (moving on to ambulant care and home care) and the number requiring more assistance will increase (patients coming from nursing homes), the demand for care per patient per day will increase.

3.2.4 Measures required

The panel was asked to state the measures from which it expected the maximum positive effect on the various aspects of RA. In most cases the members of the panel were asked to place their answers in order of priority. The members of the workshop were asked to do the same with their answers, taking into account the expected cost-benefit ratio. Where such a prioritization was possible, some variation emerged between the participants in the workshop. Different disciplines laid the emphasis on different priorities, though there was consensus that a total package of action should be taken in all fields, rather than just a small number of measures being stimulated.

Incidence

The panel was asked what fundamental research topics should be stimulated. To this end, the panel members were first asked to list those areas in which scientifically important advances were *expected*. They were also asked whether these advances would lead to primary prevention and a fall in incidence before the year 2005, or whether it was only the knowledge of the topic which would increase, without any direct consequences for primary prevention and incidence being realized. (The latter aspect could well have an effect on secondary prevention, i.e. prevention of irreversible damage). Table 3.7 summarizes the topics listed, and gives the percentage of respondents expecting positive results for each topic. The measure of desirability of stimulating research into these topics corresponds with the order of priority presented in this table.

Table 3.7 Expectations of the panel concerning the effect of fundamental research. The percentage of respondents is shown (N = 15)

	Type of advance		
Research topic	Breakthrough	More knowledge only	None
Immune response mechanism	47	47	7
Genetics	27	53	20
Viruses and bacteria	27	27	47
Other factors such as nutrition, hormones, psychosocial factors	0-10	30	60-70

The respondents expect an increase particularly in the knowledge of the immune response mechanism and of genetic aspects, partly as a result of developments in connection with AIDS research.

When panellists were asked which aspects should be the subject of specific research, they listed the expression processes of the RA-predisposing genes under the influence of exogenous factors, and the relationship with the disturbed (auto-)immune response.

Although a considerable proportion of the Delphi panel expects that advances before 2005 will lead to primary prevention and a decrease in the incidence of RA, there was unanimous agreement in the workshop that the panel had been too optimistic. According to the participants in the workshop, primary prevention will not be possible before 2005

Provision of care

The panel was asked which developments or measures in the area of care provision should receive *additional stimulation.* Twelve developments were listed by more than 45% of the panel, in the following order of priority:

1. Additional (in-service) training of general practitioners in rheumatic diseases.
2. Intensification of the collaboration between primary and secondary health care, partly on the basis of a referral policy and feedback reporting.
3. The setting up of rheumatology teams with a rheumatologist as the central "figure".
4. More rheumatologists.
5. More attention for socio-medical matters and psychology in training care providers.
6. Increased quality of existing hospital rheumatology units.
7. Expansion of home help.
8. Deployment of a hospital and community-based nurse working from the secondary health care system (rheumatology centre) and acting as an intermediary between primary and secondary health care.
9. More/better information and education provided by rheumatologists and paramedics to RA-patients and their partners/families.
10. The institution of ergotherapy in primary health care.
11. Deployment of district nurses with special attention for rheumatic diseases.
12. More/better information and education provided by rheumatologists and general practitioners to employers, medical examiners, Joint Medical Service physicians and Industrial Insurance Administration Office doctors.

Clear priority was given to additional (in-service) training of general practitioners in rheumatic diseases. The setting up of rheumatology teams and the appointment of more rheumatologists were mentioned virtually exclusively by respondents working in secondary health care.

A variety of answers was received on the question of how in-hospital rheumatology care should be organized. For example, 16% of the respondents would like to see an increase in the present number of specialized rheumatology hospitals, 39% would like to see no change and 26% favour a reduction; 19% have no opinion on this question. There was a similar variety of opinion, even within disciplines, on the organizational structure and the desired number of rheumatology departments in teaching and general hospitals. There was, however, a preference among respondents employed in the primary health care sector and in outlying hospitals for a reduction in specialized rheumatology hospitals and an expansion of the number of rheumatology departments in general hospitals, while respondents employed in teaching hospitals or specialized rheumatology hospitals expressed a preference for an expansion of the rheumatology departments in teaching hospitals. A desire for the expansion of the number of specialized rheumatology hospitals was only expressed by respondents working in these institutions.

On some, more concrete measures, however, there was a broader consensus. For example, 65% of the respondents felt that specialized rheumatology hospitals and separate rheumatology departments should be *attached to teaching centres or "top hospitals"*. this would improve the level of care, enabling the specialized facilities to be maintained.

48% of the respondents considered that the *contacts* between specialized rheumatology hospitals *and primary health care* should be expanded and supported. The rheumatology hospitals should provide more support for primary health care, while their direct provision of care to the patient could decrease. This could be achieved, for example, through a hospital and community-based nurse who could provide or initiate the necessary specialized care at home. The patient, following a short period of additional expert help, would then be able to manage once again for some time with self-care, informal care and primary health care.

45% of the panel considered that there is a need for more *multidisciplinary collaboration*, for example by the combining of rheumatology and rehabilitation.

There was less consensus on some other measures. For example, 32% of the panel felt that the present level of care should be *maintained*. RA demands specific care for which contributions from several disciplines need to be called in so that attention can be given to more than one aspect of the disease. The same percentage (32%) would like to see a better *spread*, with each region having a centre in which expertise is concentrated, as long as the number of beds is large enough to enable specialized care to be provided as well. Collaboration with other centres would be desirable here.

29% of the panel felt that the *quality* of specialized rheumatology hospitals needs to be *increased in all cases*, irrespective of whether the number of rheumatology hospitals increases, decreases or remains the same. 26% of the respondents felt that rheumatology hospitals should switch to a partially *ambulant* mode of operation.

13% would like to see the *abolition* of specialized rheumatology hospitals. They see these hospitals as expensive, isolated institutions where multidisciplinary diagnosis and treatment falls short of the requirements. There are problems in achieving a satisfactory link with other essential medical and rehabilitation facilities. According to this group of respondents rheumatology services should not be provided in isolation from other care.

29% of the panel are in favour of the expansion of *rheumatology departments in teaching hospitals*, partly in connection with the training of students, etc. According to 26% of the respondents there should be an increase in the number and quality of the *rheumatology departments in general hospitals*, though it would then be necessary for care-providers to be given specific training in rheumatic diseases. The number of rheumatology hospitals could then be reduced or remain static.

It can be concluded that there is a fairly wide difference of opinion among the members of the panel regarding the structure of in-hospital rheumatology services. There is even a lack of consensus within the different disciplines. The present and future role of specialized rheumatology services needs to be studied further according to the participants in the workshop.

A prerequisite for optimum care in outpatient clinics is that patients are able to consult rheumatologists regularly. The seven rheumatologists on the panel were therefore asked how many times a year an "average" RA-patient who is currently being treated by a rheumatologist should be examined, and what the minimum length of such an examination, excluding discussion, administration, etc., should be. The medians of the responses were five times per year (the minimum and maximum values were 3.5 and 8 respectively), and 20 minutes per examination (minimum and maximum 10 and 30 minutes respectively). The respondents felt that the time spent with the patient should be 100 minutes per year (minimum and maximum values 53 and 180 minutes, respectively). It should be noted that the frequency and length of consultations depend heavily on the severity of the disease.

Other aspects of optimum rheumatological services are currently being examined in a needs assessment study which is being undertaken by the Catholic University of Brabant in collaboration with the University Hospital of Groningen.

Quality of life

The following social factors were listed by the panel as deserving more attention from government or social groupings (e.g. professional groups) in order to promote as far as possible the psychosocial component of the quality of life for a large group of RA-patients (the points are listed in order of priority):

1. Employment opportunities.
2. Application of the Handicapped Employees (Employment) Act.
3. Modifiable dwellings in city centres.
4. Accessibility of buildings and public transport.
5. Public information on rheumatic diseases.
6. Subsidies for adaptation of dwellings and for appliances.
7. Development and availability of appliances.
8. Discussion groups/patient networks.
9. Acceptance of handicapped people by society.
10. Informal care (i.e. greater attention for the overloading of this network).

A number of social developments which were not listed are expected to develop "autonomously" (cf. section 3.2.3), without requiring additional attention. Examples include an increase in the capacity of RA-patients to perform general daily activities, an increase in the awareness of the disease and in patient assertiveness, and an increase in self-care.

It is striking that there are a number of aspects which the panel members do not expect to develop as "autonomous trends", but to which they also do not give high priority as requiring stimulation. These aspects include living according to a set regimen, problems concerning sickness absence, incapacity for work and unemployment, fear of handicaps, dependence on others, becoming lonely and isolated, social contacts, sport and play opportunities and the additional costs of RA.

Life expectancy

58% of the respondents hold the view that it is not possible to increase the life expectancy of RA-patients (further) beyond the extension which is already expected (see section 3.2.2. "Life expectancy"). 33% hold the opposite view. The measures proposed by this 33% are as follows:

1. Lower toxicity of the medication (listed by 33% of the panel).
2. Early, lasting inhibition of infections (listed by 25%).
3. Obtaining more insight through research into genetic predisposition and the influence of exogenous factors (listed by 13%).
4. Improved care-provision with regard to pain, discomfort and psycho-social aspects.
5. Improved planning and urban development to reduce the number of accidents.

4 FUTURE SCENARIOS: Possible situations in the year 2005

4.1 Introduction

This chapter describes four future scenarios based on the baseline study, the Delphi study and the workshop discussions. In the first instance it was necessary to put together a systematic package of different types of scenarios, each containing sufficient detail to allow qualitative assessment or quantitative calculation of their consequences for the year 2005.

The following four future scenarios were produced:

I. The demographic scenario, in which all parameters except demographic developments were kept constant; the computation on this scenario provides insight into the effects of demographic changes which are also present in the other scenarios (section 4.2).

II. The reference scenario, which contains the most likely developments according to the Delphi respondents, but which leaves out the demographic developments (section 4.3).

III. Two alternative scenarios, which give an impression of the possible breadth of variation of future developments (section 4.4).

IV. The policy scenario. This scenario examines the possibilities open to the government and other organizations for optimizing the chances for a favourable scenario. This scenario is discussed predominantly in qualitative terms (section 4.5).

The object of the first three exploratory scenarios is to give an indication of the boundaries within which future developments may take place. The scenarios give a partially quantitative, though mainly qualitative description of what developments are possible on the basis of various assumptions relating to the number of rheumatoid arthritis patients, the number and severity of articular features and extra-articular manifestations, quality of life and medical consumption. The policy scenario examines the possibilities of influencing the developments.

4.2 Demographic scenario (I)

The computation of the effect of demographic developments in the period 1990-2005 is roughly based on the mean variant of the CBS population forecast. The change in the size of the population in the Netherlands in 2005 as compared with 1990 in terms of age and sex can be read off from Figure 4.1.

Figure 4.1 Population size in the Netherlands in 1990 and 2005 by age and sex

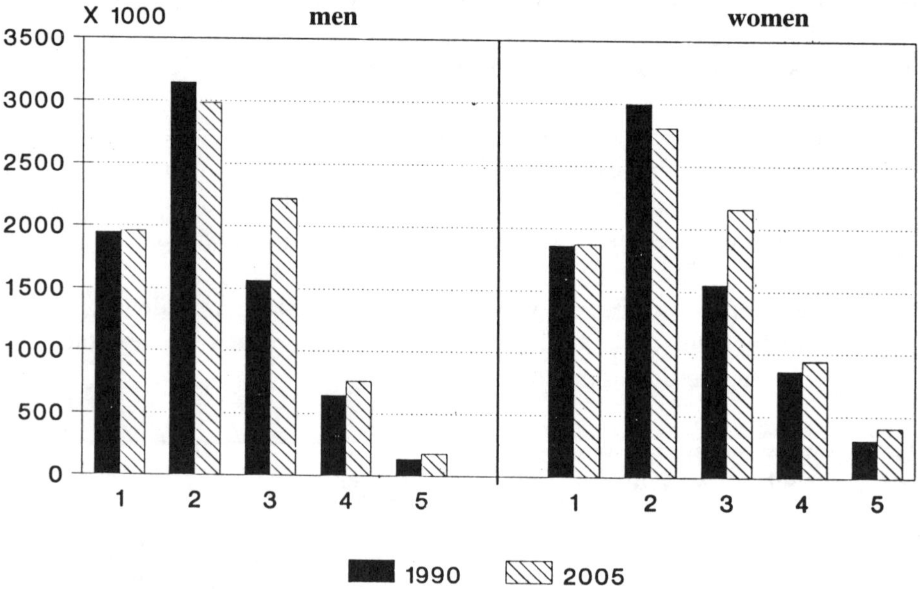

1 = age 0-19
2 = age 20-44
3 = age 45-64
4 = age 65-79
5 = age ≥ 100

The figure shows the following:

1. Overall there is an increase of 8.9% for men (from almost 7.4 million in 1990 to approximately 8.1 million in 2005) and 8.1% for women (from approximately 7.6 million in 1990 to around 8.2 million in 2005), with an average increase of 8.5%. For the sake of clarity, no column for the total figures have been included.

2. In the age category 0-19 there is virtually no increase in the size of the population (0.6% for both men and women), while in the age category 20-44 there is actually a decrease (5.2% for men and 6.4% for women).
3. From the age of 45 onwards there is a continual increase in the size of the population, with the peak being in the age group 45-64 (42.0% for men and 39.2% for women). This development is the result of the post-war baby boom.
4. There is a relatively large increase in the population in the 65-79 age group (17.9% for men and 9.5% for women), and this increase is even more pronounced in the age category 80+ (31.8% for men and 33.1% for women). This fact will not have a major influence on developments in the absolute number of patients in the population as a whole, however, since the number of people in the age category 80+ is small.

The effect of these demographic changes on the number of patients with RA (section 4.2.1) and medical consumption due to RA (section 4.2.2) in the period 1990-2005 will be discussed below, in sections 4.2.1 and 4.2.2 respectively.

4.2.1 Number of patients with rheumatoid arthritis in the period 1990-2005

As stated earlier (section 2.2.1.2), the modelling of possible future developments in the number of patients with rheumatoid arthritis (RA) is based on both the prevalence found in the Zoetermeer Epidemiological Preventive Survey (EPOZ) (1) and on the prevalences registered at the Nijmegen University General Practitioners Institute (NUHI) (2). The epidemiological study gives an insight into the prevalence of RA among the population, while the morbidity surveillance provides insight into the occurrence of cases of RA known to general practitioners.

This distinction is necessary, since the take-up of health care facilities by patients known to the physician/general practitioner cannot simply be equated to the take-up of facilities by the additional patients traced in an epidemiological study. A complicating factor is that the patients known to the physician/general practitioners do not also appear *per se* in the epidemiological study; in fact, in the Zoetermeer survey this was the case only 60% of the time (see section 2.2.1.2).

The calculations of the anticipated number of patients with RA in the period 1990-2005 are based on the assumption that the number of patients with RA per 1,000 inhabitants of the Netherlands (the prevalence) will remain constant over time for each age and sex category. Multiplying the age and sex-specific prevalence by the expected number of inhabitants in the period up to 2005 in the category in question therefore enables the influence of demographic developments on the change in the absolute number of patients to be calculated. This is referred to as the **static** or **equilibrium model**.

In contrast to the situation with diabetes mellitus (3), it is not possible to construct a dynamic model for rheumatoid arthritis which takes account both of an age and sex-specific inflow of new patients and an outflow of known patients. Reliable data on the inflow (incidence) and outflow (mortality and recovery) of patients with RA are not available.

Figure 4.2 Number of patients with rheumatoid arthritis in the period 1990-2005 on the basis of the EPOZ (from the age of 20) and the NUHI (all ages and including ankylosing spondylitis) according to the static model

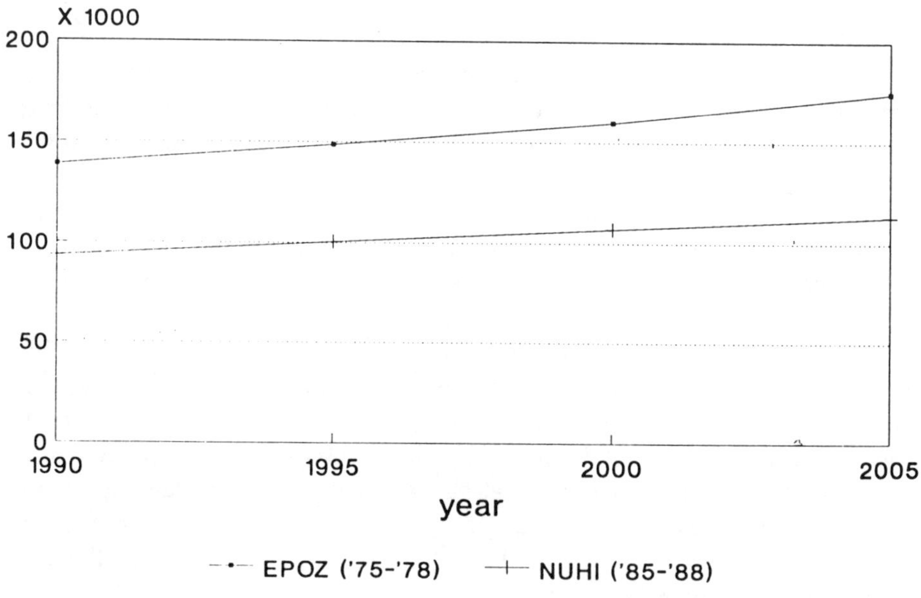

Figure 4.2 shows the increase in patients with RA in the period 1990-2005 according to the static model, both for the number of patients found in the **epidemiological study** (EPOZ) and for the number as known to general practitioners according to the **morbidity records** (NUHI). Tables 2.1 and 2.3, respectively, show the prevalences on which the calculations are based.

It is apparent from Figure 4.2 that the absolute number of patients with RA is increasing in both cases. The increase in RA-patient numbers is relatively larger on the basis of the EPOZ (25.8%) than according to the NUHI (21.0%).

In contrast to the morbidity records, the epidemiological study did not cover the age category up to 20 years old. However, for the interpretation of the increase in the number of patients according to the EPOZ compared to the NUHI this is of little relevance, since the number of RA-patients under the age of 20 is small compared to the total number of patients (1.9%) and the increase in the numbers of this section of the population is only 0.6% over the next 15 years (see Figure 4.1).

The trend in the absolute number of patients is not the same for all age groups, and there are also sex-related differences. The calculation are therefore age and sex-specific. The respective bases for the calculations are the prevalences of RA as found in the EPOZ (see Table 2.1) and registered in the NUHI (Table 2.3). The initial prevalences were related to age groups as small as possible in the calculations. However, the results are given only in four and five age-groups, respectively (Figure 4.3 and 4.4).

Although there are differences of detail, there are strong correspondences between Figure 4.3 and 4.4. On the basis of the demographic scenario, the number of female RA-patients in particular will increase over the next 15 years. On the basis of the EPOZ, this increase is approximately 25,500, compared with approximately 10,000 for men; on the basis of the NUHI, the female and male increases are approximately 12,000 and 7,500, respectively. The largest increase is in the age group 45-64, something which was to be expected on the basis of Figure 4.1.

Figure 4.3 Change in the number of patients with rheumatoid arthritis in the period 1990-2005 by age and sex, on the basis of the prevalences in the EPOZ*

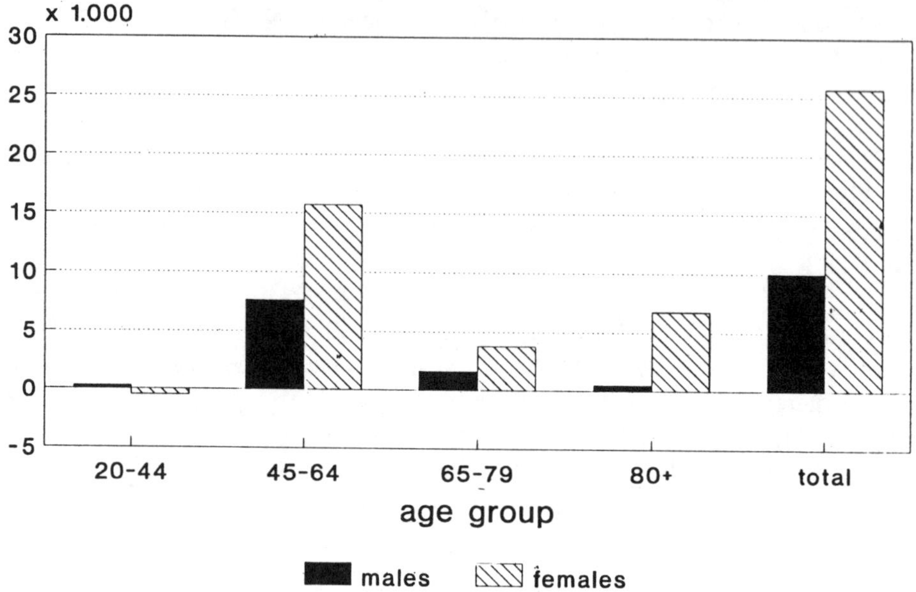

* Annex 5 (Table 1) gives the figures for patients with rheumatoid arthritis by age and sex for the years 1990 and 2005, as well as showing the percentage change.

There is relatively little difference between the percentage increases for men and women (see Annex 5). On the basis of the EPOZ the increase figure for men and women is approximately 26%, on the basis of the NUHI approximately 23% for men and 20% for women. Related to age, the relative increase is largest in the age group 45-64 (post-war baby boom) followed by the 80+ age group (ageing).

Different population forecast

In computing the demographic projections, a population forecast was chosen which corresponds with the mean variant of the CBS population forecast. However, it would also be possible to choose different population forecasts. This section will look briefly at the sensitivity of the results if different baseline values are adopted for the population forecast.

Figure 4.4 Change in the number of patients with rheumatoid arthritis (including ankylosing spondylitis) in the period 1990-2005 by age and sex, on the basis of the prevalences in the NUHI*

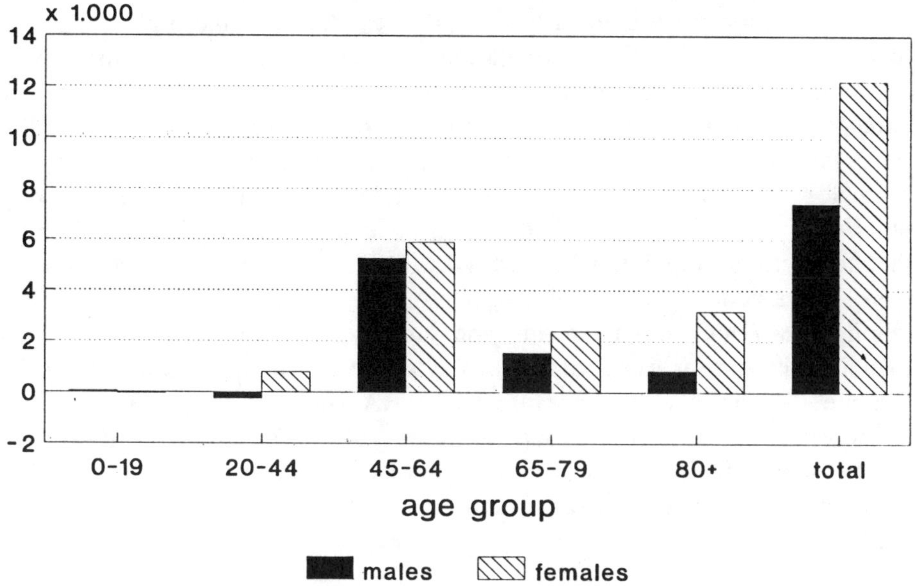

* Annex 5 (Table 2) gives the figures for the number of patients with rheumatoid arthritis (including ankylosing spondylitis) in the period 1990-2005, specified according to age and sex, as well as the percentage change.

The high variant of the CBS population forecast puts the population in 2005* at over half a million higher than the mean variant (3.5% more men, 3.4% more women); the low variant estimates half a million less (4.4% fewer men, 4.1% fewer women).

On the basis of the NUHI figures, the sensitivity of the results to different population forecasts proves to be slight. According to the high variant the number of male RA patients in 2005 will increase by an extra 2.9% and the number of female patients by an extra 1.6% compared with the mean variant. The low variant estimates the number of male and female RA-patients at 2.1% and 2.4%, respectively, lower than the mean variant. The

* The CBS does not provide age-specific forecasts for the low and high variants for 2005, so the average of the figures for 2010 and 2000 has been used here.

percentage change in the number of men and women with RA is always smaller than the change in the population.

The explanation for this must be sought in the fact that the high, mean and low variants of the CBS population forecast show mutual differences particularly in respect of the birth-rate and the expected average life expectancy. Apart from variations in the predicted size of the total population, this leads to differences between the forecasts particularly in the projected number of young people (aged 0-19) and the number of very elderly people (80+). Both relatively and, in particular, in absolute terms, the population in the high and low variants will deviate most strongly from the mean variant in the age group 0-19. The prevalence of RA among men and women in this age group is low (Table 2.3), and this explains the insensitivity of RA to changes in the population forecast. Despite the fact that the prevalence of RA (including ankylosing spondylitis) is high in the age group 80+ (see Table 2.3), this has little effect on the sensitivity to changes in the population forecast, due to the small number of people in the Netherlands in the 80+ age group (compared to the 0-19 age group).

4.2.2 Medical consumption

With regard to future demand on care facilities as a result of RA, it can be stated that, if the pattern of need and the care policy were to remain unchanged, medical consumption will grow in line with the number of patients. On the basis of the demographic scenario, this means a growth of approximately 21% in medical consumption by 2005 compared with 1990. For those forms of care where there is a high level of consumption among the older age groups (e.g. outpatient care and nursing home care), however, the ageing phenomenon will lead to an additional increase in demand (the number of patients over the age of 80 is likely to increase by approximately 30%). Although no reliable data are available, it is reasonable to assume that this also applies to district nursing care and home help. Unfortunately, through lack of data it is not possible to indicate the absolute extent of medical consumption in 2005.

4.2.3 Conclusion

The calculations clearly show that the expected demographic changes will lead to a rise in the prevalence of the number of (known) RA-patients in the year 2005 compared to 1990. An estimate based on the NUHI data and calculated using the static model shows an increase of 21% in the absolute number of *known rheumatoid arthritis patients* in 2005. Approximately 8.5% of these will be attributable to the population growth (16.3 million people in 2005 compared with 15.0 million in 1990), and 12.5% to a changed population composition (ageing). On the basis of the EPOZ figures, the static model shows an increase of 25.8%. At the same time it is apparent from the NUHI data that in calculating the absolute number of patients up to 2005, the sensitivity of RA (including ankylosing spondylitis) to different population forecasts is low.

It is not clear how realistic these percentage increases are, since the static model takes no account of the continuing effects of past trends. The literature contains indications of a decrease in annual incidence (see 2.4.1), and the possibility therefore cannot be ruled out that the percentage increases have been overestimated. It was not possible to construct a dynamic model for RA which takes account of these past trends, due to a lack of reliable data on the inflow of new patients (incidence) and the outflow of known patients (mortality/recovery).

If only demographic changes are incorporated in the model, medical consumption **as a result of** RA increases in line with the number of patients - though the age-dependency of medical consumption means it increases more strongly for some care facilities, such as outpatient care and nursing home care. Although no reliable data are available, it is reasonable to assume that this also applies to district nursing care and home help. The absolute level of the medical consumption in the year 2005 cannot be predicted with any certainty, however.

4.3 Reference scenario (II)

The reference scenario is based on the **main forecast** of the respondents in the Delphi study. Where necessary, slight adjustments were made on the basis of the results of the workshop. This scenario is based on the respondents' personal perceptions of expected autonomous developments and future government/non-government policies. To a significant extent these forecasts are based presumably on developments (which take place separately from government-controlled developments) in health care with regard to research, prevention and treatment of RA. The respondents were asked in the Delphi study to indicate these future developments, *assuming a constant population size and structure.*

On the basis of the results of the Delphi study and the workshop (see Tables 3.1 and 3.2) the reference scenario for RA can be described as follows. Given a stable population, the incidence of RA up to the year 2005 is not expected to change. Against this, RA will be diagnosed in an increasing number of as yet undiagnosed patients. The life expectancy of RA-patients is expected to increase slightly more rapidly than that of the population in general. A decline is expected in the incidence and severity of a number of features associated with RA. The number of iatrogenic complications, by contrast, may well increase. There will be a slight improvement in quality of life. An increase is forecasted in the number of patients receiving primary and outpatient care, while the percentage receiving care in hospitals, specialist centres, nursing and rest homes will remain stable or show a slight fall. The amount of care needed by RA-patients receiving primary, secondary and tertiary care is likely to remain unchanged or to increase slightly.

The most important arguments produced by Delphi respondents in support of the forecast changes will be briefly discussed below.

Incidence will remain unchanged because no change is expected up to 2005 in the genetic predisposition to RA or in exposure to primary causal agents (such as viruses and bacteria), which may be responsible for the onset of RA.

The forecasted increase in the percentage of patients actually diagnosed will come about, in the respondents' view, as a result of greater expertise, particularly of general practitioners, an increase in patient assertiveness, better awareness among the "public" and increased accessibility to specialists. Improved, more refined and new diagnostic methods could also be significant here.

The forecasted developments with regard to the articular features of RA include a reduction in the incidence and severity of pain, function impairment and deformities. Early diagnosis of RA, early initiation of an adequate therapy and better-informed patients are put forward as the reasons for this. The result will be a decrease in the level of dependence on others.

In addition to the articular features of RA there are also the extra-articular manifestations to consider. The predicted fall in the incidence and severity of one of these, amyloidosis, is the result of early diagnosis, following which more aggressive treatments will be administered at an early stage. No changes are expected in the incidence or severity of the other extra-articular manifestations.

It is not unlikely that there will be an increase in the incidence of iatrogenic complications as a result of the earlier administering of more aggressive medicinal therapy, and also as a consequence of the use of medicines with which little experience has yet been gained. The more frequent use of immunosuppressive therapy and the development of resistant hospital infections during joint operations, etc. may lead to an increase in the risk of infection as an iatrogenic complication. Consequently, it is important to remain alert to the occurrence of iatrogenic complications.

The quality of life is expected to improve slightly. On the one hand this can be attributed to the improvements described above with regard to articular features and extra-articular manifestations. On the other hand, improvements are also expected on a psychosocial level, with the most important developments being the potential improvements in the availability of appliances and facilities which will enable patients to function more independently.

According to the respondents, the additional increase in life expectancy will result from earlier recognition of RA, which will enable the improved therapy to be initiated at an earlier stage of the disease.

The increasing concentration on primary health care is mainly attributed to an anticipated improvement in the organization and content of primary health care. There will be an increase in outpatient care because fewer patients will be admitted to hospital and because improved diagnosis will result in more referrals to specialists. The shift towards outpatient treatment will lead to a fall in the percentage of RA-patients receiving in-hospital care. This in turn will lead to an increase in the demand for care per patient for those who do receive hospital care, since those remaining will be relatively serious patients.

The expected improvement in the organization and content of primary health care will lead to some movement away from nursing home care to primary health care. As with hospitalized patients, this will lead to an increase in the demand for care per patient in nursing homes. The percentage of patients receiving rest home care is expected to remain unchanged. On the one hand, substitution of care may mean that home care and ambulant care will be sufficient for some RA-patients. On the other hand, a proportion of the patients who would previously have entered nursing homes will in the future go to rest homes. This will lead to an increase in the demand for care per patient receiving rest home care. There was no unanimous view among the respondents regarding the direction in which the care provided by specialized rheumatology hospitals will develop over the coming years.

Calculations

The reference scenario combines both favourable and unfavourable trends. According to the main forecast of the experts, the ultimate result of these trends is unchanged incidence and an additional increase in life expectancy of one year over the period 1990-2005 compared with the population in general. Through the lack of reliable epidemiological data it is not possible to include the consequences of such an increase in life expectancy in calculating the expected number of RA-patients up to 2005. On the basis of the model adopted in the scenario study for diabetes mellitus, however, it is unlikely that such a change in life expectancy would have a significant effect on this calculation.

By contrast, it is possible to quantify the effect of the increase forecasted by the respondents in the percentage of **diagnosed** patients. The respondents expect that 60% of all patients will have been diagnosed in 2005, compared with 50% in 1990. This projection takes no account of the expected increase on the basis of improved, more refined and new diagnostic methods, since it was not possible to express these factors numerically.

The NUHI figures give an impression of the number of (diagnosed) patients with RA who are known to general practitioners. According to these data, there were approximately 93,500 patients with RA who were known as such to their general practitioner in 1990. If the rate of diagnosis were to remain unchanged at 50%, this would lead to a figure of approximately 113,000 in 2005 (demographic scenario). If on the other hand a

60% rate of diagnosis in 2005 is assumed, this figure will rise to around 135,500 patients known by their general practitioners to be RA-patients. This is an additional increase of 22,500 patients on top of the demographic scenario, or an increase of approximately 45% compared with the number of patients in 1990 (see Table 4.1). It is highly likely that this additional increase relates to patients with less serious forms of RA.

Table 4.1 Number of patients with rheumatoid arthritis (including ankylosing spondylitis) (x 1,000) known to their general practitioners in 1990 and 2005 with an unchanged (demographic scenario) and a changed (reference scenario) rate of diagnosis

Scenario	1990	2005	1990-2005 Increase absolute	%
Demographic scenario*	93.5	113	19.5	21
Reference scenario*	93.5	135.5	42	45

* Unchanged rate of diagnosis of 50%
** Changed rate of diagnosis, from 50% in 1990 to 60% in 2005

A degree of caution is needed when interpreting the increase in the rate of diagnosis, in view of the wide spread of answers by the respondents regarding the current rate of diagnosis and what that rate will be in 2005. Within the EPOZ, too, it is impossible to state with any certainty what percentage of RA-patients are known to their general practitioners. According to this survey, the percentage lies anywhere between 20 and 75% (see pp. 47 and 48).

4.4 Alternative scenarios (III)

The alternative "autonomous" scenarios are intended to serve as contrasts to the reference scenario. While the latter reflects the most likely developments according to the experts, the alternative scenarios show extreme variants, which are just about possible. They thus give an indication of the possible variation within the forecasts.

In terms of content, the alternative scenarios are formulated on the basis of an analysis of the current situation and the results of the Delphi study. They are based on ideas emerging from the study group, the Scenario Committee and the participants in the workshop.

In selecting alternative scenarios it is important to choose those which on the one hand have a high impact, and on the other are not regarded as a likely autonomous development - hence the term "low probability, high impact" scenario. Those developments and measures were selected which could have a high impact on the incidence of RA and life expectancy, the occurrence and severity of articular features and extra-articular manifestations of RA, quality of life or medical consumption.

Only two types of alternative scenario are described here: a case-finding scenario and an austerity scenario. It proved impossible to produce a quantitative effects estimate for both types of alternative scenario, and this will therefore be discussed in detail only for the case-finding scenario (active detection of as yet undiagnosed RA-patients). In addition, a qualitative description will be given of the possible consequences if there are major cutbacks in health care and in society as a whole over the coming year (austerity).

Case-finding

In this context, case-finding is understood to mean the active detection of as yet undiagnosed RA-patients. These may for example be patients who display RA-like symptoms on an intermittent rather than a continuous basis (i.e. at intervals). There is an important task here for the general practitioner, who is in the best position to draw together "isolated" episodes of RA-like symptoms and leading to a suspicion of the presence of RA.

Case-finding is of great importance if there is a serious degree of underdiagnosis and in situations where adequate treatment, applied early, could halt the progression of the disease. The fact that there is indeed a considerable degree of underdiagnosis has already been stated in section 4.3. According to the Delphi respondents the rate of diagnosis in 1990 is 50%. A recently published article surveys the importance of early diagnosis combined with adequate treatment (including information, exercises and medication) as a means of preventing irreversible damage (5). The importance of this is also clearly underlined by the Delphi respondents.

This alternative scenario is based on the assumption that in the most extreme case in the coming 15 years, case-finding will lead to early diagnosis of all patients with RA. The rate of diagnosis in 2005 is then 100%, which means that in the year 2005 there will not be approximately 135,500 known RA-patients (based on the reference scenario, see section 4.3), but approximately 226,000 - an increase of 142% over the number of patients in 1990. The comment was made during the workshop that 100% case-finding in 2005 is very extreme. Just feasible, but still extreme, is a diagnosis percentage of 90%; this would represent an increase in the number of patients compared to 1990 of 118%.

Austerity scenario

The austerity scenario sketches the consequences of a number of economy measures which may be adopted in times of economic recession. RA-patients are a vulnerable group, since they are not only dependant on health care which is both quantitatively and qualitatively good and accessible, but are also in a disadvantaged position in other areas of society. This section therefore looks not just at economy measures in the field of health care, but also at measures taken in other areas.

In the event of insufficient availability of health care in the future (as a result of restriction, stabilization or inadequate growth in the availability at macro-level), or of reduced accessibility of the facilities (due to limitation of the package of services), a proportion of the RA-patients will be unable to obtain adequate care, and some may even receive no care at all. Other economic cutbacks, such as the building in of financial thresholds for eligibility for health care facilities, will also result in certain groups of RA-patients losing their access to the care facilities they need. A survey of RA-patients who are either being treated by specialists (6) or are members of the Netherlands Rheumatism Association (the "Reumabond") (7) shows that, even now, they face additional annual costs ranging on average from approximately NLG 1,500 (6) to NLG 1,750 (7), including travel costs, costs of domestic/nursing help, footwear/clothing, appliances and special facilities. The economy measures described above would lead to these groups falling further behind financially, with resultant reduced welfare and greater pressure on the informal care network. At a later stage, however, the economies could actually result in additional health care costs if (a proportion of) the RA-patient group, due to a lack of care, develops a form of RA which is sufficiently serious to make admission to the care system unavoidable.

Economies outside the health care sector - for example, a reduction in the level of social benefits - can also have extremely adverse consequences for RA-patients. Studies have shown that a large proportion of RA-patients depend on these benefits (6,7). Financial constraints in areas such as the supply of appliances and (building) adaptations, and cutbacks in job incentive schemes for the partially disabled (such as the Handicapped Employees (Employment) Act) affect the RA-patient group.

Economy measures in respect of facilities which (a large proportion of) RA-patients *have to* use often not only affect the welfare of RA-patients, but also have an adverse effect of the level of morbidity, and perhaps even on the mortality rate. Measures of this sort put patients in an even more disadvantaged position.

Unfortunately, the situation outlined above is not entirely improbable. Several of the measures described have in fact already been announced (e.g. economies in physiotherapy), and other similar plans are currently being worked out (particularly in the context of changes to the system, the Drugs Compensation Scheme, householder's levy for home adaptations, etc.)

4.5 Policy scenario (IV)

This section looks at the policy scenario. A general policy objective is to achieve the WHO targets for chronic diseases, which specify a reduction of 10% in the level of invalidity by the year 2000. This general objective has also been formulated to match the Dutch situation in the draft Discussion Document on Health Policy (8, 9).

This objective needs to be made more specific, since it is not clear from the WHO target whether the aim should be a 10% reduction in the total population or "per patient"; nor is the term invalidity or impairment described further. The most obvious approach for chronic diseases, in view of the influence of ageing, is to formulate the target "per patient". For RA, for example, the policy objective could be to achieve a 10% reduction per

RA-patient by the year 2000 in the occurrence of articular features and extra-articular manifestations of RA. According to the Delphi panel, a reduction in the occurrence and severity of articular features is to be expected, though the same does not apply to extra-articular manifestations, with the exception of amyloidosis. To the extent that reducing the articular features and amyloidosis promotes the quality of life, the envisaged 10% reduction also represents a (partial) objective in relation to the quality of life.

The policy scenario has been selected by choosing those aspects in respect of which the Delphi respondents, the Scenario Committee and the study group feel that the initiation and stimulation of measures will enable the problem of RA to be tackled most effectively over the coming 15 years. There are three central themes in the policy scenario: prevention, medical care and social functioning (see Table 4.2).

Table 4.2 Policy scenario themes

a Prevention	- Fundamental research
b. Medical care:	- Expansion of care - Health care innovations
c. Social functioning	

Before looking in more detail at this policy scenario for RA, the extent to which the scenario corresponds to or differs from the scenarios as formulated by the TNO Rheumatic Committee for Rheumatology Research (CR-TNO) in the report "Towards a new Juncture" ("Naar een nieuw Tijdsgewricht") is described (10). This report formulates objectives with respect to (the financing of) **rheumatology services, education in rheumatology** and **rheumatology research**. Three scenarios were drawn up, which share the common feature that the infrastructure must be improved by reducing the dependence on collection-box funds and providing a system of structural funding. Scenario I "Down to the bone" ("Tot op het bot") is a modest, conservative and consolidating scenario. Scenario II "In motion" ("Bewegen") provides for a gradual growth of all aspects of (university) rheumatology. For the care of rheumatism, this means that the present shortage of available care should be attuned to the demand for care, while account needs to be taken of the increasing need for care. In addition, education and research need to be stimulated. Scenario III "Towards a new Juncture" attempts on top of this to produce practical solutions to the problems of the accessibility of care. In presenting its report, the TNO Rheumatic Committee for Rheumatology Research states that one of the results of the implementation of this scenario could be a reduction in the number of Invalidity Insurance Act cases due to rheumatic diseases (Rasker, personal communication).

It is striking that in spite of the different angles of approach (the TNO Rheumatic Committee for Rheumatology Research took as its starting point improvement of the research infrastructure, while the Scenario Committee started from the expected developments in numbers of patients and the burden on the care system), the elements care, education and research, as set out in Scenario III of the TNO Committee report are also included among the various themes of the policy scenario for RA drawn up by the Scenario Committee for Chronic Diseases (see Table 4.2). All the themes, in the view of the participants in the workshop, should receive attention. The shortfall in the available care and the increasing need for care are dealt with as part of the theme "medical care" under the heading "Expansion of care" (Table 4.2). The accessibility of care with respect to this theme is discussed under "Health care innovations", as is the importance of education. The theme "prevention" highlights the importance of scientific research. Additional recommendation for future scientific study are also given in section 5.5.

As well as these correspondences, there are also some points of difference. The scenarios produced by the TNO Rheumatic Committee for Rheumatology Research relate to rheumatology as a whole, including RA, and cover the period 1990-1995. The scenarios are geared towards the implementation of concrete plans. The desired expansions are formulated in quantitative terms, and the financial consequences and organizational framework are described. However, the social functioning of rheumatic patients as such is less explicitly stated in these scenarios. The Scenario Committee, by contrast, felt compelled to devote separate attention to this matter in its policy scenario for RA-patients. In addition, the Scenario Committee's scenarios cover a longer period, namely 1990-2005. By illustrating the growth in the number of patients and the demand on care in the various scenarios, a number of possible policy choices - and the associated costs - are implied. The demographic scenario entails the least sharp rise in costs, while the reference scenario is likely to involve more costs (as a net result of economies and incentives); implementation of the policy scenario is the most expensive option.

The various themes from the policy scenario for rheumatoid arthritis are discussed in more detail below.

a. Policy geared to prevention

There is still insufficient understanding of the causes of RA to allow successful preventive measures to be taken. On the other hand, this understanding is increasing, and research into the causes of RA therefore needs to be strongly encouraged, particularly in those areas where experts feel that substantial progress is possible. A big increase in this understanding is considered particularly possible with respect to the immune response mechanism, and the relationship between this mechanism and genetic predisposition to RA and primary causal agents such as viruses and bacteria. It is unlikely, however, that it will be possible to use the increased knowledge of the immune response mechanism before 2005 for primary prevention of RA, with a resultant noticeable decrease in incidence before then; the effects of this increased knowledge are likely to become apparent only in the longer term.

By contrast, it is highly likely that improved secondary prevention, defined here as the prevention of irreversible damage, for example to the joints, will be possible earlier than this. Increased knowledge of the immune mechanism will allow the immune system of RA-patients to be influenced in a more targeted way using medication. This will make it possible to exert an influence on the progression of RA, thus avoiding a great deal of suffering. Information on the effectiveness of this influence will have to come mainly from longer-term patient-related scientific research.

b. Medical care

An outline is given here of developments and measures which lead to an improvement in RA-care. The purpose of the measures is twofold: to produce an improvement in the welfare of RA-patients, combined with a decrease in morbidity and mortality. A distinction is made between expansion of care and health care innovations.

Expansion of medical care

If RA-care is to be adequate in the future, the first requirement is that the level of facilities is expanded. Four reasons are given below for the need for this expansion of care. In most cases it proved impossible to quantify precisely the care availability needed.

1. In the first place, the level of available care needs to be expanded to take account of demographic developments (see demographic scenario). If the need for care is to be met, the level of care facilities will have to be increased by an average of 21%. As stated earlier, the ageing of the population will lead to a relatively stronger increase in the number of older RA-patients. This means that those care facilities which are utilized particularly by older RA-patients (e.g. outpatient and nursing home care, and possibly also district nursing and home help services) will have to be expanded to a relatively greater extent.
2. It is likely that more as yet undiagnosed RA-patients will be detected (see reference scenario), leading to an increase in the number of RA-patients not of 21%, but of 45%. This additional increase will relate mainly to patients with milder forms of RA. In order to meet this additional increase in the need for care (which comes on top of the increase due to demographic developments), the number of general practitioners and rheumatologists, in particular, will need to be increased.
3. As already described in the reference scenario, a shift is expected to take place from nursing home and hospital care to ambulant primary and secondary health care (specialists, general practitioners, district nurses). A number of reasons can be put forward for this, such as the general policy of substitution, improvements in out-of-hospital RA-care, etc. This change in the need for care, too, will necessitate a change in the level of facilities available in the future (additional expansion of ambulant primary and secondary health care).
4. The fourth reason for expanding the amount of care is bound up with the present problems surrounding the level of care available for RA. The number of rheumatologists (and also their distribution throughout the country) is felt to be inadequate at the moment to be able to guarantee good RA-care. An expansion is not only necessary for the purposes of direct patient care, however, but is also a condition for expanding the tasks of rheumatologists in terms of consultation, coordination of care and providing additional training to other care-providers. At the request of the Ministry of Health, the Catholic University of Brabant is currently carrying out a joint study with the State University

of Groningen to determine how many rheumatologists are needed now and in the longer term in order to meet the need. This study is looking not just at RA, but covers a much wider range of rheumatoid diagnoses.

At the start of 1991 the Ministry of Health commissioned another study, carried out by the Hospital Facilities Council, into the need for a review of the standard range of care provided by orthopaedists (12). This study showed that the present number of orthopaedic specialists is inadequate to meet the present and future demand for care. It was calculated that in 1999 there would be a need for an extra 30 full-time orthopaedists in order to reduce waiting lists. The waiting list problem is due primarily to the number of specifically orthopaedic operations, such as joint-replacement surgery for RA-patients and others. The norm established in 1986 of one orthopaedic surgeon per 52,000 inhabitants is too low; the Council considers that in the period 1990-1995 a norm of one surgeon per 45,000 inhabitants is needed. Up to 1995 the number of orthopaedists needs to be increased by another 13, while for the longer term (up to the year 2000) a care outreach of one surgeon per 40,000 inhabitants may well be necessary. The Council also points out that the solution must be sought not only through the bringing in of more orthopaedists; financial difficulties also require attention (limited hospital budgets).

Another problem relates to the shortage of professional workers within the home care system (family carers, district nurses and health visitors). Measures to improve home care are not only important for the RA-patients themselves, but also reduce the pressure on the informal care network. According to the Delphi panel, this pressure is currently already at a maximum, and threatens to increase still further. The problem is also not simply the shortage of these care-providers; the accessibility of these types of care is also inadequate, due among other things to financial strictures and strict rules relating to the content of care.

Health care innovations

There are many possible ways of improving RA-care. The most important measures and developments are described here. Health care reforms divide into two components: a content component and an organizational component.

The most important measure as regards the *content* component of the care provision involves improving the expertise of the care-providers with respect to RA. As well as improving the basic training, other ways must be developed of increasing the expertise of care-providers already working in the field, for example through additional training. Some kind of "bonus system", which rewards the following of additional training courses, is desirable.

The main target of improving expertise is the general practitioner; if he or she has more expertise, it is highly likely that RA-patients will be diagnosed at an earlier stage, enabling treatment to begin earlier, which in turn will enable the course of the disease to be influenced. Another target within the primary health care system, however, are district nurses, who need to obtain greater knowledge and experience regarding RA. Rheumatology district nurses have an important role to play in improving training here. The present trend, whereby reorganization of home nursing has led to enforced despecialization of district nurses, is seen as an undesirable development. What is required is the deployment of home-care nurses who have a specific interest in rheumatic diseases, including RA. An important requirement here is that the development of expertise is accompanied by the opportunity to acquire sufficient practical experience with RA-patients.

However, it is not only the professional development of care-providers in the primary health care system which requires attention. Rheumatologists, too, require additional training in certain aspects of RA (including the diagnosis and treatment of system disorders in RA-patients). A point worth looking at here is whether it would not be better to treat RA-patients on the basis of guidelines (protocols). Before such a move could be implemented, however, thorough research would be needed into these protocols, and consensus would have to be reached regarding their content.

In addition to knowledge regarding recognition of RA-symptoms, diagnostic techniques and treatment, the extra (in-service) training also needs to devote (more) attention to socio-medical matters and psychological aspects. This would probably enable the care-providers to provide more effective information and support to RA-patients and their families which, in addition to improving the psychosocial care, could also lead to a greater role for the RA-patient him or herself in the treatment process ("shared care").

An important *organizational* problem in RA-care has to do with the "barriers" between primary and secondary health care. Attempts need to be made to improve the cooperation and coordination between primary and secondary health care providers working in the care of rheumatoid arthritis. This could be promoted by setting up "rheumatology teams" with a rheumatologist as the central figure, supported by a rheumatology consultant (hospital and community-based nurse), who would act as an intermediary between primary and secondary health care. In addition to tasks involving direct patient care, the rheumatologist (together with the rheumatology consultant) would also act as a case manager, would have a consultative function, would stimulate additional training, etc. An approach such as this offers many advantages: the RA-care provided at the various locations in the health care system would be more mutually complementary, general practitioners would become more expert, individual GPs and rheumatologists would be more aware of each others' capabilities and limitations, etc. It should be borne in mind here that a rheumatology team such as this would not be designed to focus exclusively on RA-patients, but also on a number of other rheumatological disorders.

In its report "Towards a new Juncture" published by the TNO Rheumatic Committee for Rheumatology Research (10) recommends a similar approach to rheumatological care. The increase in expertise and improved cooperation between the various care-providers would enable RA-patients to be diagnosed at an earlier stage, enable treatment to begin earlier, mean that the treatment is qualitatively better and enable more attention to be devoted to psychosocial support. According to the Scenario Committee, the general practitioner, in addition to the early detection of patients, has a further twofold function here. He or she would have an important task in respect of all RA-patients in providing psychosocial support and detecting symptoms of RA and side-effects of medication, etc.; in addition, for those RA-patients who do not use secondary medication and whose disease is in a stable condition, the general practitioner could also (temporarily) act as the treating physician. It is very important for this approach that explicit guidelines are drawn up for the coordination of care between the rheumatologist and the general practitioner (protocol development).

c. Social functioning

As already indicated in the alternative austerity scenario, RA-patients are currently still in a disadvantaged position socially. Besides the fact that their disease makes them dependent on medical care, their employment opportunities are more restricted; they have to enter into extremely complex and lengthy procedures in applying for appliances and home adaptations; public and other buildings, usually make no allowances for the more disabled RA-patients; and society still shows too little understanding to RA-patients and handicapped people in general.

As a result of their disease some RA-patients are less capable of performing work, and this may result in sickness absence, incapacity for work or unemployment. For the patient, however, this is an extremely undesirable situation and, theoretically at least, if the proper adaptations were carried out and use was made of existing legislative possibilities, also an unnecessary situation. This could be avoided to some extent through better enforcement of the Handicapped Employees (Employment) Act and by giving more and better information to employers, personnel assistants, medical examiners, Joint Medical Service and Industrial Insurance Administration Office doctors regarding the capabilities and limitations of RA-patients, and regarding the available appliances, adaptations, etc.

There is also a good deal of room for improvement in the area of appliances and adaptations. Besides the fact that RA-patients are often inadequately informed of what is available here, the application procedures are extremely complex and lengthy. More flexible financial arrangements for ergotherapy, and enabling ergotherapists to provide care in the patient's home situation, would be major improvements in this respect. It is also highly recommended that the mass of regulations and procedures surrounding applications for adaptations should be simplified and made more flexible, so that "customized care" can be offered. The financial help should be such that the costs do not form a barrier preventing patients from obtaining the necessary appliances/adaptations. In addition, municipal (re)development plans, the construction/alteration of buildings, public transport, etc., need to make greater allowance for less able persons (for example, sufficient modifiable dwellings in the vicinity of shopping centres).

The other area for attention within this theme relates to influencing public opinion regarding rheumatic diseases (including RA) and the handicapped. Information can play an important role here, provided this is given in a structured and professional manner.

4.6 Conclusions

On the basis of the demographic developments (**demographic scenario**) the static computational model indicates that the total number of *known patients* with rheumatoid arthritis (including ankylosing spondylitis) (NUHI) in the Dutch population will be almost 21% higher in 2005 than in 1990.

This increase may be an *overestimate* since it takes no account of the continuing effect of past trends, whereas there are indications for a *decrease* in incidence in the period prior to 1990 (see section 2.4.1). Construction of a dynamic model, which does take account of past trends, proved not to be possible for RA due to a lack of reliable data concerning the inflow of new patients (incidence) and outflow of known patients (death/recovery).

Calculations based on the static model show an increase in total medical consumption as a result of RA which is of the same order as the increase in the number of patients. As a result of the age-dependence of the medical consumption, there is a *stronger increase* in the *consumption of a number of facilities*, such as outpatient care and nursing home care. Although no reliable data are available, it is reasonable to assume that this also applies to district nursing care and home-help services.

The most likely development up to the year 2005 according to the Delphi respondents, the so-called **reference scenario** indicates a *bigger increase* than the demographic scenario in the number of diagnosed patients. This is due to an expected increase in the rate of diagnosis. The respondents expect that 60% of patients will be diagnosed in 2005 compared with 50% in 1990. As a result, the increase in the number of known patients will not be almost 21% compared with 1990, but around 45%.

On the other hand, no change is expected in the incidence in the next 15 years, while life expectancy will probably increase by (only) one year compared with the population in general. On the basis of the model used for diabetes mellitus, it can be projected that such a change in life expectancy will not have a significant effect on the likely number of RA-patients in 2005.

According to the experts on the Delphi panel, there will be some decrease in a number of articular features and extra-articular manifestations which an average RA-patients develops during his or her lifetime. As a result of this, and also as a consequence of improvements on a psychosocial level (partly with regard to the availability of appliances and facilities which will make it easier for RA-patients to function independently), the quality of life is expected to increase somewhat.

Beyond this, it is expected that both the percentage of RA-patients receiving care and the demand for care per patient receiving care within the primary health care system and at outpatient clinics will increase. The percentage of patients receiving care in hospitals and nursing homes is expected to decrease, while the demand for care per patient will increase. The percentage of patients receiving care in rest homes is likely to remain stable, with demand for care per patient increasing. There was no consensus regarding the direction in which the care provided by specialized rheumatology hospitals will develop in the coming years.

A combination of the "most probable" developments obviously has a smaller chance of becoming reality in precisely that form than each individual forecast development. A whole series of different developments can be imagined around the reference scenario, with the **alternative autonomous scenarios** as the "extremes". Two types of alternative autonomous scenario were developed in this project, a case-finding scenario and an austerity scenario. These alternative scenarios make it clear that different assumptions regarding (autonomous) future developments can lead to quite different situations in the year 2005.

The **policy scenario** makes it clear that experts see various possibilities for changing the situation favourably with respect to incidence, articular features and extra-articular manifestations of RA, and the quality of life of RA-patients. Fundamental research into the causes of RA, expansion of care, health care innovations (including education) and attention for social functioning are expected to have important positive effects. Recommendations for future scientific research are dealt with separately in section 5.5. It is noteworthy that the policy scenario for RA largely corresponds with Scenario III "Towards a new Juncture" constructed by the TNO Rheumatic Committee for Rheumatology Research for the whole range of rheumatological disorders (including RA).

5 CONCLUSIONS: PRIORITY AREAS FOR POLICY

5.1 Introduction

This chapter indicates a number of priority areas for policy according to the Scenario Committee. First a brief explanation is given of the priorities as indicated in the policy scenario, following which a cohesive policy is formulated. Finally, the chapter considers the deficiencies in the provision of information and the importance of scientific research as a support for policy.

5.2 Setting priorities

Policy geared to prevention

There is still insufficient understanding of the causes of RA to allow successful preventive measures to be taken. On the other hand, this understanding is increasing, and research into the causes of RA therefore needs to be strongly encouraged, particularly in those areas where experts feel that substantial progress is possible. A big increase in this understanding is considered particularly possible with respect to the immune response mechanism, and the relationship between this mechanism and genetic predisposition to RA and primary causal agents such as viruses and bacteria. It is unlikely, however, that it will be possible to use the increased knowledge of the immune response mechanism before 2005 for primary prevention of RA, with a resultant noticeable decrease in incidence before then; the effects of this increased knowledge are likely to become apparent only in the longer term.

By contrast, it is highly likely that improved secondary prevention, defined here as the prevention of irreversible damage, for example to the joints, will be possible earlier than this. Increased knowledge of the immune mechanism will allow the immune system of RA-patients to be influenced in a more targeted way using medication. This will make it possible to exert an influence on the progression of RA, thus avoiding a great deal of suffering. Information on the effectiveness of this influence will have to come mainly from longer-term patient-related scientific research.

Expansion of medical care

High priority must be given to the expansion of medical care, for a number of reasons. In the first place the ageing of the population and the increase in the rate of diagnosis will lead to a rise in the number of patients with RA in the coming years. Ageing is expected to lead to an increase of 21% in the number of diagnosed patients in the period 1990-2005 (demographic scenario). If the future need for care is to be met, the level of care available will have to grow in line with this need. As a result of the ageing process, the older patient group will increase relatively more strongly, leading to a need for additional expansion of those forms of care which are directed particularly at this group of patients, (outpatient care, nursing home care and - though no reliable data were available - district nursing care and home-help services).

If the expected increase in the rate of diagnosis is also taken into account, the number of RA-patients will increase by approximately 45% (reference scenario). The additional increase probably relates to patients with less severe forms of RA, and this is expected to lead to a particular increase in the demand placed on outpatient clinics, general practitioners and the use of medicines.

Independent of the increase in the number of patients, the percentage of patients receiving care, particularly primary health care and outpatient care, is also expected to increase, as is the demand for care per patient receiving these types of care (reference scenario).

A fourth reason for expanding care is bound up with the present problems within RA-care, where the amount of care currently available does not correspond with the demand for that care. The shortfall applies particularly to specialized rheumatological care. The extent of this shortfall is currently being studied by the Catholic University of Brabant in collaboration with the State University of Groningen; this study looks not only at RA, but also at other rheumatological diagnoses. The report published in early 1991 by the Hospital Facilities Council also described a shortfall in the area of orthopaedics (section 4.5) (1).

Health care innovations

Given the present problems facing RA-care, attention also needs to be given to improving the quality of the care. Measures to improve this quality could probably produce visible results relatively quickly. In particular, more attention needs to be given to increasing the expertise of care providers, especially general practitioners (among other things by improving basic training, developing post academic training programmes, which could perhaps be made compulsory). There is also a need to increase the knowledge of other care providers (such as district nurses, home helps and rheumatologists) in certain areas. The additional training should include explicit attention for socio-medical and psychological aspects. An important aspect of increasing expertise is to ensure that care providers obtain sufficient experience in dealing with the problems of patients with RA.

On an organizational level, attention needs to be given to improving the collaboration between primary and secondary health care with respect to RA-patients. A solution could be provided by the setting up of "rheumatology teams" in which a rheumatologist and a rheumatology consultant (hospital and community-based rheumatology nurse) occupy a central role. As well as providing (part of) the treatment and supporting RA-patients, these persons would also function as "case managers", coordinating the care of individual patients, and would also have a consultative function for other care providers (transfer of expertise).

Social functioning

As RA-patients are currently still in a disadvantaged position, it is also important to stimulate measures to improve their social functioning. Employment opportunities for RA-patients could be improved by more effective enforcement (with sanctions) of the Handicapped Employees (Employment) Act; increasing and improving the information given to employers, personnel officers, medical examiners, Joint Medical Service and Industrial Insurance Administration Office doctors could also make a contribution here.

Other measures which would improve the social functioning of RA-patients include better access to ergotherapists, simpler and more flexible rules covering ergotherapy and application procedures for appliances and adaptations, constructing "adaptable" buildings, etc. Influencing public attitudes to rheumatic diseases (including RA) and handicapped people (for example through information), could play an important role here.

Implementing measures in the above areas demands powerful support from the government, health insurers and professional organization.

5.3 Formulation of a coherent policy

The main impulses for new developments in the field of rheumatology have come from within the care system itself and from scientific research (see also section 5.5), although some impulse has also come from the government.

Within the field of health care there are several associations active in the area of rheumatic diseases, including RA. The National Rheumatism Fund and the Netherlands Association for the Control of Rheumatic Diseases (NVRB) can be seen as a functional unit whose objective is to promote the fight against rheumatic diseases in the Netherlands. The financial resources of the National Rheumatism Fund are made available to the NVRB for fighting rheumatic diseases in the Netherlands. The most important areas in which the Association is active are as follows:

1. Providing support for scientific research.
2. Providing financial help to individual rheumatology patients;
3. Implementing an extensive recreation programme.
4. Subsidizing rheumatology patient associations.
5. Providing information.

Another body active in this field is the Rheumatic-Diseases Research Committee of the Health Research Division of TNO (Netherlands Organization for Applied Scientific Research), which coordinates research into rheumatic diseases. This committee, which was originally set up by the Ministry of Health, also acts at the request of the NVRB as an advisory body with regard to the scientific research which is subsidized by that body. Other organizations include the Dutch Federation of Associations of Patients with Rheumatic Diseases, which has 16,500 members from 92 local patient associations and which publishes the monthly journal "In Beweging" ("On the Move"); the Netherlands Society of Rheumatologists; the Netherlands Association of Rheumatoid Surgery (NVRC), known until 18 March 1991 as the Netherlands Rheumatoid Arthritis Surgical Society (NERASS); the Netherlands Association of Rheumatology Nurses and Carers; and the National Working Group for Physiotherapy in Rheumatic Diseases.

The tripartite consultations between the NVRB, the Netherlands Federation of Associations of Patients with Rheumatic Diseases and the Netherlands

Society of Rheumatologists (founded in 1983) bring together the various parties for the purpose of exchanging information, consultation and setting joint policy.

In contrast to diabetes mellitus, and to a greater extent than CNSLD, rheumatic diseases have attracted regular government attention in recent years. Thus, for example, on the basis of recommendations issued by the Science Policy Advisory Council (1983, (2)) and the Health Council (1985, (3)) in the Health Research Promotion Programme in 1985 (SGO, (4)), high priority was assigned to research into rheumatic diseases. Subsequently this was developed as the first component in the Promotion Programme, in which respect a programme was drawn up for the years 1986-1990 (see section 5.5). In addition, the Rheumatic Diseases Policy Document which was published as one of the annexes to the 1989 draft Discussion Document on Health Policy published also devoted separate attention to rheumatic diseases (5) and formulated a number of policy proposals. The "Chronic Diseases" scenario study is a further policy initiative by the government in the field of rheumatic diseases, and especially RA.

In its policy document "Working towards Innovations in Health Care", the present government has announced a number of important policy proposals, including giving priority to chronic diseases. The Chronic Diseases Policy Memorandum, which was submitted to the Dutch Lower House in early 1991 (6), identifies a number of problem areas for a range of chronic diseases, including RA. The policy memorandum was formulated on the basis of discussions held with various organizations. The problem areas, which particularly reflect the view of patient organizations, form the "input" for the National Committee for the Chronically Ill, which was founded in mid-1991 and which has both an advisory role and a number of executive tasks. The Health Policy Document submitted to the Lower House in the autumn of 1991 continues the themes initiated by the draft Discussion Document on Health Policy (7).

Of importance is the fact that the government is developing an integral policy plan for chronic diseases in consultation with those working in health care. Rheumatic diseases, including RA, should be given an important place in these discussions in view of the scale and severity of the problem. The research policy needs to be looked at in detail in the policy plan as many questions remain unanswered. In addition, a strong stimulus for research should be given now; within the framework of the elaboration of the report "Towards a new Juncture", RA health care providers are clearly working on this (see sections 4.5 and 5.5).

5.4 Improving the provision of information

To a greater extent than in the scenario study "Accidents and Traumatology" the Chronic Diseases Scenario Committee was hampered by a lack of reliable data on RA. This made the construction of even a general picture of the terrain a difficult task. The same also applied to diabetes mellitus and CNSLD, though the problem was even more pronounced in the case of RA.

Where no data were available, a choice had to be made in the background chapter (Chapter 2) between presenting general impressions and leaving out estimates altogether. The latter alternative was chosen, preference being given to a conservative report based on empirical data, since this was a first detailed presentation of the field, and it was therefore important that this be as firmly based possible.

An important register, the Standard Diagnosis Register of Rheumatic Diseases (SDR) was begun in 1977 by the TNO Rheumatic Committee for Rheumatology Research. This register provides information relating mainly to outpatient rheumatological care.

There remain significant shortcomings in the recording of RA, however. The most notable of these are:

1. A lack of recent, reliable (trend) data on the incidence and prevalence of RA in the population. The most recent study was the EPOZ, which was conducted in 1975-1978.
2. A lack of reliable data on the incidence of RA in general practice. The populations studied are too small to enable well-founded statements to be made on this matter.
3. In so far as they are available, the data on the incidence of articular features and extra-articular manifestations of RA are inadequate, particularly as regards their development in individual patients.
4. There is a lack of reliable (trend) data on medical consumption as a result of this disease. As far as consumption has been recorded it tends for a number of reasons to suffer from underreporting (e.g. in the LMR/SIG).

5. There is a lack of reliable (trend) data on mortality as a result of RA. There are reasons to assume underreporting in the CBS cause-of-death statistics.

In contrast to diabetes mellitus and CNSLD, it was felt that in view of the greater lack of reliable information there was little point in a detailed discussion of the costs associated with RA-care both now and over the next 15 years. Further research is definitely needed here.

The setting up of the continuous surveillance projects to chart the extent of the RA problem is therefore a first priority for policy formulation.

5.5 Importance of scientific research

Scientific research is of great importance for policy development in the longer term. This applies even more emphatically to the research policy of the Netherlands Association for the Control of Rheumatic Diseases and other organizations which carry out or subsidize research in this field (Ministry of Health, Ministry of Education and Sciences, Ministry of Social Affairs and Employment and the pharmaceuticals industry).

The main impulses for new developments in scientific research in rheumatology have come from the field of health care itself. The TNO Committee for Rheumatology Research has played a key role here, coordinating the scientific research since 1971. Thanks to this committee, a number of effective alliances have been created such as the Standard Diagnosis Register of Rheumatic Diseases and the Rheumatology Standardization Working Group.

New insights into the RA problem can be expected from current or imminent studies. The following projects are worthy of mention:

1. Studies subsidized by the Netherlands Association for the Control of Rheumatic Diseases/National Rheumatism Fund (see 1989 annual report).
2. Rheumatology research carried out via the Health Research Promotion Programme.
3. A study to assess the need for rheumatologists, carried out by the Catholic University of Brabant in collaboration with the State University of Groningen.

4. The Multiple Echelons Rheumatology Study (ROME), carried out by the TNO Committee for Rheumatology Research. This is a fact-finding study into the referral patterns and problem areas which exist in the cooperation and coordination between the various care providers.
5. European Research on Incapacitating Diseases and Social Support (EURIDISS). This project focuses primarily on research into the importance of social support and networks for the functioning of those with chronic diseases, especially RA-patients.
6. The "National Study of Diseases and Treatments in General Practice" and the monograph "Chronic Diseases" carried out by the Netherlands Institute for Primary Health Care Research (Utrecht).

One important function of the Chronic Diseases scenario study is to map the "blank spots" in the research. Precisely because a lack of information was observed in so many areas, it is possible to generate a large number of ideas for research. This in turn makes it necessary to devise a coherent package of research topics and thus place the RA research policy within a clearer framework. The TNO Committee for Rheumatology Research, in its report "Towards a new Juncture" (8), also identifies a number of problem areas with respect to scientific research. These problem areas are incorporated in the research topics listed below. We shall confine ourselves to the most important topics:

Monitoring:

1. Conducting an epidemiological **population study.** This would provide insight into the present extent of RA (making comparison possible with previous epidemiological surveys). In addition, the patients known to general practitioners could be compared with those newly discovered as a result of the population study. The study would need to be longitudinal in order to allow the determinants for the prognosis of RA to be analyzed. It would also need to be set up along the same lines as other international studies in this field.
2. The setting up and continuation of continuous monitoring projects in **a large number of general practices** needs to be coupled with scientific research in order to provide a reliable insight into the trends in RA and the (trends in the) development of articular features, extra-articular manifestations and medical consumption. The aim must be to enable an overall assessment of the degree to which the RA problem is increasing or decreasing. Here again, alignment would have to be sought with international studies in this field.

3. There should be a commitment to increasing the number of rheumatologists taking part in the SDR so that **outpatient care** can be charted at a national level. Serious consideration should also be given to integrating this register with the SIG's outpatient surveillance system (POLIS).

Prevention:

1. Research into the causes of RA needs to be strongly encouraged (see section 4.5, prevention scenario), with a view to both primary and secondary prevention.

Treatment and care:

1. Research into the (problems of) accessibility of rheumatology services, i.e. professional help by rehabilitation physicians, physiotherapists, ergotherapists, rheumatology consultants, general practitioners, area and district nurses and home helps (this is currently being investigated for rheumatologists and a study has just been carried out for orthopaedists).
2. Research into the help actually provided by the patient's immediate support circle and other volunteers, as well as research into the consequences of the provision of that help by those close to the patient (e.g. overburdening).
3. Research into the accessibility of adaptations and appliances (including in the work situation).
4. Research into the effects, accessibility and quality of the information provided through patient associations, Health Information and Education (GVO) consultants and professional carers.
5. Research into the quality of life of RA-patients. This should include an investigation into optimal methods of coping with the disease. Aspects of the quality of life should be taken into account in the evaluation of particular developments and measures.
6. Research in the area of medication. This should be seen as an extension of the research into the causes of RA. A better understanding of the immune mechanism will enable treatment to be administered in a more targeted way. In addition research is needed into the long-term effects of medication.
7. Research into the role of physiotherapy. Are there particular categories of RA-patients for whom a particular therapy is effective, and what is that effect?
8. Research into the present and future role of specialist rheumatological care.

The TNO Committee for Rheumatology Research notes that the training of research workers who concentrate on basic and patient-related research is currently one of the greatest problem areas, as is the career planning of these research workers, given the short-term nature of the majority of research projects.

A special recommendation made to the Steering Committee on Future Health Scenarios is that the RA scenario study might be continued in the form of an update study (which would not need to be so time-intensive), so that a document will become available in a few years' time covering the developments which have taken place with regard to RA. On the basis of the new data it would then be possible to assess whether the actual developments had turned out differently from those projected in the reference scenario. The scenario which most closely matched the actual situation would then provide an impression of the possible consequences, thus creating a basis for adjustment of the policy aims.

5.6 Conclusion

Although chronic diseases have much in common, thereby enabling an overall chronic diseases policy to be formulated (9), there is also a marked need for specific policies related to each disorder. This report accordingly focuses on these specific aspects.

The "RA" scenario study is intended as a contribution to the planning of long-term policy by the Dutch government with respect to this health problem. The study provides policy-makers with insight into a number of quantitative and qualitative relationships at the present time and into the consequences of various scenarios. Taken as a whole, these indicate the limits within which future developments are likely to take place.

The study makes it clear that policy-makers can **not** act on the assumption of favourable "autonomous" developments. An adequate quantitative and qualitative response to the growing number of RA-patients will require major efforts on the part of the government, care providers, patients and society in general. The same applies to an even greater degree to reducing the extent of the problem through prevention and making up the shortfall of care in the field of rheumatic diseases.

REFERENCES

Chapter 1

1. Ontwerp-Kerndocument Gezondheidsbeleid. Doelgericht veranderen voor de jaren 1990-1995 (Draft Discussion Document on Health Policy. Purposive change in the years 1990-1995). Ministry of Welfare, Health and Cultural Affairs, Rijswijk, 1989.
2. Nota 2000: over de ontwikkeling van gezondheidsbeleid: feiten, beschouwingen en beleidsvoornemens (Policy Document 2000: On the development of health policy, facts, considerations and policy intentions). Parliamentary Proceedings, Lower House, 1985-1986 session, 19500 nos. 1-2, Rijswijk, 1986.
3. Werken aan Zorgvernieuwing. Actieprogramma van het beleid voor de zorgsector in de jaren negentig (Actions for innovation in health care). Parliamentary Proceedings, Lower House, 1989-1990 session, 21545 no. 1, Rijswijk, 1990.
4. Notitie Chronisch-Ziekenbeleid. Chronische patiënten buiten spel (Memorandum on Chronic Diseases Policy. Chronic Patients on the Sidelines). Ministry of Welfare, Health and Cultural Affairs. Parliamentary Proceedings, Lower House, 1990-1991 session, 22025, no. 1, Rijswijk, 1991.
5. Stuurgroep Toekomstscenario's Gezondheidszorg. Ongevallen in het jaar 2000 (Steering Committee on Future Health Scenarios. Accidents in the year 2000). Bohn, Scheltema en Holkema BV, Utrecht, 1988.
6. Berg J van den, Bos G.A.M. van den: Het (meten van het) voorkomen van chronische aandoeningen, 1974-1987 (Incidence and measurement of chronic diseases). Maandbericht Gezondheid, CBS, 1989, nr. 3, 4-11.
7. Davidse W, Water HPA van de, Vaandrager GJ. Selectie van chronische ziekten voor scenario-onderzoek. Methodologische keuzeproblemen (Selection of chronic diseases for scenario research. Methodological problems of choice). Med Cont, 1988, 43, 493-4.
8. Davidse W, Water HPA van de, Vaandrager GJ. Toekomstscenario's chronische ziekten - vooronderzoek (Future scenarios on chronic diseases - preliminary research). Leiden, Nederlands Institute for Preventive Health Care, 1987.
9. Steering Committee on Future Health Scenarios. Chronic Diseases in the year 2005. Part 1, Scenarios on diabetes mellitus 1990-2005. Bohn, Scheltema & Holkema, Utrecht/ Antwerp, 1990.

10. Steering Committee on Future Health Scenarios. Chronic Diseases in the year 2005. Part 2, Scenarios on CNSLD 1990-2005. Bohn Stafleu van Loghum, Houten/Antwerp, 1990.
11. Steering Committee on Future Health Scenarios: Scenario's in de volksgezondheid. Inleiding in de methodiek van de STG (Public health scenarios. An introduction to the methods of the STG). Van Arkel, Utrecht, 1989.

Chapter 2

1. Cats A, Putte LBA van de. Reumatische ziekten (Rheumatic diseases). In: Ottolander GJH den (red.). Interne Geneeskunde (Internal Medicine), 9th revised impression. Bohn, Scheltema & Holkema, Utrecht, 1989: 343.
2. Gewanter HL, Roghmann KJ, Baum J. The prevalence of juvenile arthritits. Arthritis Rheum 1983; 26: 599-603.
3. Ropes MW, Bennett GA, Cobb S, Jacox R, Jessar RA. Revision of diagnostic criteria for rheumatoid arthritis. Bull Rheum Dis 1958; 9: 175-176.
4. Kellgren JH. Diagnostic criteria for population studies. Bull Rheum Dis 1962; 12: 291-292.
5. Bennett PH, Burch TA. New York Symposium on population studies in the rheumatic diseases; new diagnostic criteria. Bull Rheum Dis 1967; 17: 453-458.
6. Arnett FC, Edworthy SM, Bloch DA. The American Rheumatism Association 1987 revised criteria for the classification of rheumatoid arthritis. Arthritis Rheum 1988; 31: 315-324.
7. Epidemiologisch Preventief Onderzoek Zoetermeer (EPOZ) (Zoetermeer Epidemiological Preventive Survey), fifth progress report, Volume 4, "Rheumatic Diseases". Erasmus University Rotterdam, Institute of Epidemiology, 1979.
8. Continue Morbiditeits Registratie Nijmeegs Universitair Huisartsen Instituut (Continuous Morbidity Surveillance Project, Nijmegen University General Practitioners Institute), 1985-1988. Data supplied on request. Nijmegen, 1990.
9. Den Oudsten SA, Planten O, Posthuma EPS. Longitudinal survey of RA in an urban district of Rotterdam. In: Bennett PH, Wood PHN (eds). Population studies of the rheumatic diseases. Excerpta Medica Foundation, Amsterdam, 1968.

10. ICHPPC-e-defined. International Classification of Health Problems in Primary Care. Oxford, Oxford University Press, 1983.
11. Gall EP. General features of rheumatoid arthritis. In: Schumacher HR, Gall EP (eds). Rheumatoid Arthritis. An illustrated guide to pathology, diagnosis and management. 1988: 1.21.
12. Netherlands Institute for Primary Health Care Research (NIVEL). National study. As yet unpublished provisional data supplied on request. Utrecht, 1991.
13. Vakgroep Huisartsgeneeskunde, Rijksuniversiteit Groningen. Data supplied on request, Groningen 1990.
14. Short CL, Bauer W. The course of rheumatoid disease in patients receiving simple medical and orthopaedic measures. New Engl J Med 1948: 142-148.
15. Duthie JJR, Brown PE, Truelove LH, Baragar FD, Lawrie AJ. Course and prognosis in rheumatoid arthritis: a further report. Ann Rheum Dis 1964; 23: 193-202.
16. Short CL. Rheumatoid arthritis: types of courses and prognosis. Med Clin North Am 1968; 52: 540.
17. Rasker JJ, Cosh JA. Reumatoïde artritis, een dodelijke ziekte (Rheumatoid arthritis, a fatal disease). Ned Tijdschr Geneeskd 1991; 135: 308-312.
18. Overledenen naar doodsoorzaak, leeftijd en geslacht in het jaar 1988, serie A1 (Deaths by cause of death, age and sex in 1988, series A1). Central Bureau of Statistics, Voorburg, 1988.
19. Allebeck P, Ahlborn A, Allander E. Increased mortality among patients with rheumatoid arthritis, but where RA does not appear on the death certificate. J Rheumatol 1981; 10: 301- 306.
20. Steering Committee on Future Health Scenarios. Chronic Diseases in the year 2005. Part 1, Scenarios on diabetes mellitus 1990-2005. Bohn, Scheltema & Holkema, Utrecht/ Antwerp, 1990.
21. Cobb S, Anderson F, Bauer W. Length of life and cause of death in rheumatoid arthritis. New Engl J Med 1953; 249: 553-556.
22. Reach TG. The prognosis of rheumatoid arthritis. Proc R Soc 1963; 56: 813-817.
23. Uddin J, Kraus AS, Kelly HG. Survivorship and death in rheumatoid arthritis. Arthritis Rheum 1970; 13: 125-130.
24. Isomaki HA, Mutru O, Koota IC. Death rate and causes of death in patients with rheumatoid arthritis. Scand J Rheumatol 1975; 4: 205-208.
25. Monson RR, Hall AP. Mortality among arthritics. J Chron Dis 1976; 29: 459-467.

26. Koota K, Isomaki H, Mutru O. Death rate and causes of death during a period of 5 years. Scand J Rheumatol 1977; 6: 241- 244.
27. Linos A, Worhtington JW, O'Fallon WM, Kurland LT. The epidemiology of rheumatoid arthritis in Rochester, Minnesota: a study of incidence, prevalence and mortality. Am J Epidemiol 1980; 111: 87-98.
28. Rasker JJ, Cosh JA. Cause and age at death in a prospective study of 100 patients with rheumatoid arthritis. Ann Rheum Dis 1981; 40: 115-120.
29. Vandenbroucke JP, Hazevoet HM, Cats A. Survival and cause of death in rheumatoid arthritis: a 25-year prospective follow-up. J Rheumatol 1984; 11: 158-161.
30. Mutru O, Laakso M, Isomäki H, Koota K. Ten year mortality and causes of death in patients with rheumatoid arthritis. Br J Med 1985; 290: 1797-1799.
31. Mitchell DM, Spitz PM, Young DY, Bloch DA, McShane DJ, Fries JF. Survival, prognosis and causes of death in rheumatoid arthritis. Arthritis Rheum 1986; 29: 706-714.
32. Abruzzo JL. Rheumatoid arthritis and mortality. Arthritis Rheum 1982; 25: 1020-1023.
33. Lawrence JS. Heberden Oration, 1969. Rheumatoid arthritis - nature or nurture? Ann Rheum Dis 1970; 29: 357-379.
34. Gregersen PK, Shen M, Song QL, et al. Molecular diversity of HLA-DR4 haplotypes. Proc Natl Acad Sci USA 1986; 83: 2642- 2646.
35. Zoschke D, Segall M, Dw subtypes of DR4 in rheumatoid arthritis: evidence for a preferential association with Dw4. Hum Immunol 1986; 15: 118-124.
36. Gregersen PK, Silver J, Winchester RJ. The shared epitope hypothesis: an approach to understanding the molecular genetics of susceptibility to rheumatoid arthritis. Arthritis Rheum 1987; 30: 1205-1213.
37. Winchester RJ, Gregersen PK. The molecular basis of susceptibility to rheumatoid arthritis: the conformational equivalence hypothesis. Springer Semin Immunopathol 1988; 10: 119-139.
38. Nepom GT, Byers P, Seyfried C, et al. HLA genes associated with rheumatoid arthritis: identification of susceptibility alleles using specific oligonucleotide probes. Arthritis Rheum 1989; 32: 15-21.
39. Jongh BMN de, Romunde LKJ van, Valkenburg HA, Lange GG de, Rood JJ van. Epidemiological study of HLA and GM in rheumatoid arthritis and related symptoms in an open Dutch population. Ann Rheum Dis 1984; 43: 613-619.

40. Westedt ML, Breedveld FC, Schreuder GMTh, D'Amaro J, Cats A, Vries RRP de. Immunogenetic heterogeneity of rheumatoid arthritis. Ann Rheum Dis 1986; 45: 534-538.
41. Jongh BM de, Westedt ML, Vries RRP de, Valkenburg HA, Cats A. Genetic heterogeneity of rheumatoid arthritis. Dis Markers 1986; 4: 29-33.
42. Ollier W, Venables PJW, Mumford PA, Maini RN, Awad J, Jaraquemada D, D'Amaro J, Festenstein H. HLA antigen associations with extra-articular rheumatoid arthritis. Tissue Antigens 1984; 24: 279-291.
43. Young A, Jaraquemada D, Awed J, Festenstein H. Corbett M, Hay FC, Roitt JM. Association of HLA-DR4/DW4 and DR2/DW2 with radiologic changes in a prospective study of patients with rheumatoid arthritis. Arthritis Rheum 1984; 27: 20-25.
44. Walker DJ, Griffiths M, Dewar P, Coates E, Dick WC, Thompson M, Griffiths ID. Association of MHC antigens with susceptibility to and severity of rheumatoid arthritis in multicase families. Ann Rheum Dis 1985; 44: 519-525.
45. Phillips PE. Evidence implicating infectious agents in rheumatoid arthritis and juvenile rheumatoid arthritis. Clin Exp Rheumatol 1988; 6: 87-94.
46. Venables PJW. Infection and rheumatoid arthritis. Curr Opin Rheumatol 1989; 1: 15-20.
47. Harris Jr ED. Pathophysiology and implications for therapy. N Engl J Med 1990; 322: 1277-1289.
48. Hochberg MC. Adult and juvenile rheumatoid arthritis: Current epidemiologic concepts. Epidemiol Rev 1981; 3: 27-44.
49. Kato H, Duff IF, Russell WH et al. Rheumatoid arthritis and gout in Hiroshima and Nagasaki: a prevalence and incidence study. J Chron Dis 1971; 23: 659-679.
50. Josipovic DB, Masi AT. Marked female preponderance in rheumatoid arthritis patients with younger adult onset and positive rheumatoid factor (RF) (abstract). Proceedings of XIV International Congress of Rheumatology 1977: 249.
51. Terkeltaub R. A clinical study of older age rheumatoid arthritis with comparison to a younger onset group. J Rheumatol 1983; 10: 418-424.
52. Hazes JMW. Conception, contraception and rheumatoid arthritis. Reproductive variables studied in relation to genetic susceptibility. (Thesis) Leiden University, 1990.
53. Spector TD, Hochberg MC. The protective effect of the oral contraceptive pill on rheumatoid arthritis: an overview of the analytic epidemio-

logical studies using meta-analysis. J Clin Epidemiol 1990; 43: 1221-1230.
54. Del Junco DJ. The relationship between rheumatoid arthritis and reproductive function. (Thesis) Houston, 1988.
55. Spector TD. Hormonal and reproductive factors in the aetiology of rheumatoid arthritis. (Thesis) London, 1989.
56. Medsger AR, Robinson H. Comparative study of divorce in rheumatoid arthritis and other rheumatic diseases. J Chronic Dis 1972; 25: 269-275.
57. National Center for Health Statistics. PHS, Publication No. 1000, Series 11, No. 17, Washington, U.S. Government Printing Office, 1966.
58. Korst, JK van der. Gewrichtsziekten (Articular diseases). Bohn, Scheltema & Holkema, Utrecht 1980.
59. McCormick JN, Nuki G. Diseases of connective tissues, joints and bones. In: McCleod J (ed.). Davidson's Principles and practice of medicine. 13th edn. Churchill Livingstone, New York 1981: 604-648.
60. Elst Ph. De psychische kant van reuma (The psychological side of rheumatism). In: Korst, JK van der (ed.). Reuma, part 5 in the Health Information series. Stichting Teleac, Utrecht 1983: 62.
61. McKenna F, Wright V. Pain and rheumatoid arthritis. Ann Rheum Dis 1985; 44:805.
62. Gibson T, Clark B. Use of simple analgetics in rheumatoid arthritis. Ann Rheum Dis 1985; 44:27-29.
63. Parker J, Frank R, Beck N, Finan M, Walker S, Hewett JE, Broster C, Smarr K, Smith E, Kay D. Pain in rheumatoid arthritis: relationship to demographic, medical, and psychological factors. J Rheumatol 1988; 15:433-437.
64. Rasker JJ. Reuma hebben, wat betekent reumatoïde artritis-patiënt te zijn (Having rheumatism: what it means to be a rheumatoid arthritis patient). Lederle Nederland B.V. Etten-Leur 1984.
65. Cats A, Putte LBA van de. Reumatische ziekten (Rheumatic diseases). In: Ottolander, GJH den (ed.). Interne geneeskunde (Internal Medicine). 7e revised impression. Bohn, Scheltema & Holkema, Utrecht/Antwerp 1983: 280-294.
66. Vernon-Roberts, B. Applied anatomy of joints. In: Currey, HLF (ed.). Mason and Currey's clinical rheumatology. 3rd edn. Pitman Medical Limited, Tunbridge Wells 1980: 30-63.
67. Currey HLF. Reumatologie, een beknopt overzicht (Rheumatology, a concise survey). Translated and edited by JJ de Blécourt. Stafleu, Alphen aan den Rijn/Brussels 1983.

68. Goudsmit R, Ottolander GJH den. Hematologie (Haemotology). In: Ottolander GJH den (ed.). Interne geneeskunde (Internal Medicine). 7th edition. Bohn, Scheltema & Holkema, Utrecht/Antwerp 1983: 204.
69. Decker JL, Plotz PH. Extra-articular rheumatoid disease. In: McCarty DJ (ed.). Arthritis and allied conditions, a textbook of rheumatology. 10th edn. Lea & Febiger, Philadelphia 1985: 620-642.
70. Baum J, Ziff M. Laboratory findings in rheumatoid arthritis. In: McCarty DJ (ed.). Arthritis and allied conditions, a text-book of rheumatology. 10th edn. Lea & Febiger, Philadelphia 1985: 643-659.
71. Barnes, CG. Rheumatoid arthritis. In: Currey, HLF (ed.). Mason and Currey's clinical rheumatology. 3rd edn. Pitman Medical Limited, Tunbridge Wells 1980: 30-63.
72. Zvaifler NJ. Rheumatoid arthritis: a clinical perspective. In: Lawrence RC, Shulman LE (eds.). Epidemiology of the rheumatic diseases, proceedings of the fourth international conference. Gower Medical Publishing Limited, New York/London 1984: 111.
73. Schumacher HR, Gall EP. Systemic features of rheumatoid arthritis. In: Schumacher HR, Gall EP. Rheumatoid arthritis, an illustrated guide to pathology, diagnosis and management. Gower Medical Publishing, New York 1988: 14.1-14.86.
74. Tsai J, Dalinka MK. Radiologic findings in rheumatoid arthritis. In: Schumacher HR, Gall EP. Rheumatoid arthritis, an illustrated guide to pathology, diagnosis and management. Gower Medical Publishing, New York 1988: 3.10.
75. Scott JC. Osteoporosis and hip fractures. In: Rheum Dis Clin North Am, Epidemiology of rheumatic disease, 1990; 16: 717- 740.
76. Hart FD, Rheumatoid arthritis: extra-articular manifestations. Part II. Br Med J 1970; 2: 747-752.
77. Brick JE, Brick JF. Neurologic manifestations of Rheumatologic Disease. Neurologic Clinics 1989; 7: 629-639.
78. Hamburger HL. Neurologische complicaties in de reumatologische praktijk (Neurological complications in rheumatology practice). In: Soesbergen RM, Hamelynck KJ (ed.). Conference on rheumatology surgery 1988, "Op weg naar consensus tussen reumatoloog en orthopedisch chirurg." Phizer B.V., Rotterdam 1989: 19-27.
79. Soesbergen RM, Hamburger HL. Halswervelkolom en reumatoïde artritis (Cervical vertebrae and rheumatoid arthritis). In: Soesbergen RM, Hamelynck KJ (ed.). Conference on rheumatology surgery 1988, "Op weg naar consensus tussen reumatoloog en orthopedisch chirurg." Phizer B.V., Rotterdam 1989: 79-85.

80. McGavin D, Williamson J, Forrester J, Foulds WS, Buchanan WW, Dick WC, Lee P, McSween RNM, Whaley K. Episcleritis and scleritis. A study of their clinical manifestations and association with rheumatoid arthritis. Br J Rheum 1979; 60: 192-226.
81. Schneider HA, Yonker RA, Katz P, Longley S, Panush RS. Rheumatoid Vasculitis: Experience with 13 patients and review of the literature. Semin Arthritis Rheum 1985; 14: 280-286.
82. Altena R van, Bijlsma JWJ, Kreukniet J. Pleuro-pulmonale afwijkingen bij reumatoïde artritis (Pulmonary disorders in rheumatoid arthritis). Ned Tijdschr Geneeskd 1988; 132: 1286-1291.
82. Scott DGI, Bacon PA, Tribe CR. Systemic rheumatoid vasculitis: a clinical and laboratory study of 50 cases. Medicine 1981; 60: 288-297.
83. Sokoloff L, Hough AJ. Pathology of rheumatoid arthritis and allied disorders. In: McCarty DJ (ed.). Arthritis and allied conditions, a textbook of rheumatology. 10th edn. Lea & Febiger, Philadelphia 1985: 571-592.
84. Jurik AG, Davidsen D, Graudal H. Prevalence of pulmonary involvement in rheumatoid arthritis and its relationship to some characteristics of the patients. Scand J Rheumatol 1982; 11: 217-224.
85. Roschmann RA, Rothenberg RJ. Pulmonary fibrosis in rheumatoid arthritis: a review of clinical features and therapy. Semin Arthritis Rheum 1987; 16: 174-185.
86. Medsger TA. Pulmonary manifestations of connective tissue diseases. In: Cohen AS, Bennet JC (ed.). Rheumatology and immunology (2nd edn.). Grune & Stratton, inc., Orlando 1986: 191-195.
87. Frank ST, Weg JG, Harkelroad LE, Fitch RF. Pulmonary dysfunction in rheumatoid disease. Chest 1973; 63: 27-34.
88. Dhillon V, Woo P, Isenberg D. Review, Amyloidosis in the rheumatic diseases. Ann Rheum Dis 1989; 48: 696-701.
89. Baker DG, Complications of rheumatoid arthritis. In: Schumacher HR, Gall EP. Rheumatoid arthritis, an illustrated guide to pathology, diagnosis and management. Gower Medical Publi- shing, New York 1988: 15.1-15.18.
90. Laakso M, Mutru O, Isomäki H, Koota K. Mortality from amyloidosis and renal diseases in patients with rheumatoid arthritis. Ann Reum Dis 1986; 45: 663-667.
91. Goldenberg DL. Review. Infectious arthritis complicating rheumatoid arthritis and other chronic rheumatic disorders. Arthritis Rheum 1989; 32: 496-502.

92. Mitchell WS, Brooks PM, Stevenson RD, Buchanan WW. Septic arthritis in patients with rheumatoid disease: a still under-diagnosed complication. J Rheumatol 1976; 3: 124-133.
93. Baum J. Infection in Rheumatoid Arthritis. Arthritis Rheum 1971; 14: 135-137.
94. Meijers KAE, Dijkmans BAC, Hermans J, Broek PJ van den, Cats A. Non-gonococcal infectious arthritis: a retrospective study. J Infection 1987; 14: 13-20.
95. Rijswijk MH, Houtman PM. Onderzoek naar het effect van vroegtijdige medicamenteuze interventie op de progressie van röntgenologische afwijkingen bij patiënten met reumatoïde artritis; Protocol voor de tweede fase van het onderzoek (Research into the effect of early medical intervention on the progression of radiologic disorders among patients with rheumatoid arthritis; Protocol for the second stage of the research). Groningen University Hospital, Leeuwarden Medical Centre. 1991.
96. Leufkens HGM. Pharmacy records in pharmacoepidemiology: studies on anti-inflammatory and antirheumatic drugs. (Thesis) Utrecht University, 1990: 48- 49.
97. Riel PLCM van. NSAID's: een klinisch farmacologische plaatsbepaling in de medicamenteuze behandeling van reumatische aandoeningen (NSAIDs: clinical/pharmocological positioning in the medical treatment of rheumatic disorders). Ned Tijdschr Geneeskd 1988; 132:2187-2192.
98. Central Medical Pharmaceutical Committee of the Health Fund Council. Farmacotherapeutisch Kompas 1990-1991. Amstelveen 1990: 807.
98. Putte LBA van de, Riel PLCM van. Langzaam werkende antirheumatica (Slow-acting antirheumatic drugs). Ned Tijdschr Geneeskd 1989; 133: 708-713.
99. Kremer JM. Methotrexate therapy in the treatment of rheumatoid arthritis. Rheum Dis Clin North Am 1989; 15: 533-556.
100. Trentham DE. Rheumatic therapy for the 1990s: evolution or revolution. Rheum Dis Clin North Am 1989; 15: 407-412.
101. Docken WP. Low-dose prednisone therapy. Rheum Dis Clin North Am 1989; 15: 569-576.
102. Hamelynck KJ. Algemene aspecten van de chirurgische behandeling (General aspects of surgical treatment). In: Soesbergen RM, Hamelynck KJ (red.). Conference on rheumatology surgery 1988, "Op weg naar consensus tussen reumatoloog en orthopedisch chirurg". Phizer B.V., Rotterdam 1989: 9-18.

103. Breslow L. A quantitative approach to the World Health Organisation definition of health: physical, mental and social well-being. Int J Epidemiol 1972; 1: 347-355.
104. Bell MJ, Bombardier C, Tugwell P. Measurement of functional status, quality of life, and utility in rheumatoid arthritis. Arthritis Rheum 1990; 33: 591-601.
105. Aaronson NK. Quality of life assessment in clinical trials: methodologic issues. Controlled Clinical Trials 1989; 10: 195S-208S.
106. Gough IR, Furnival CM, Schilder L, Grove W. Assessment of the quality of life of patients with advanced cancer. Eur J Cancer Clin Oncol 1983; 19: 1161-1165.
107. Rijswijk MH van, Rasker JJ. Verminderde kwaliteit van leven en levensduur bij patiënten met reumatoïde artritis (Reduced quality of life and life-expectancy among patients with rheumatoid arthritis). Ned Tijdschr Geneeskd 1991; 135: 312-313.
108. Steinbröcker O, Traeger CH, Batterman RC. Therapeutic criteria in rheumatoid arthritis. JAMA 1949; 140: 659-662.
109. Witte LP de, Tilli DJP, Ticheler AJG, Winants BAC, Horst FG van der, Linden Sj van der. Leven met een reumatische aandoening; een onderzoek naar de ervaren kwaliteit van het leven bij 372 mensen met een reumatische aandoening (Living with a rheumatic disorder; a survey among the perceived quality of life among 372 people with a rheumatic disorder). Institute for Rehabilitation Issues, Hoensbroek 1989.
110. Cornelissen PGJ. Drempelvrees; onderzoek naar de mobiliteit en sociale aspecten van reumatische aandoeningen (Qualms and inhibitions: a study of mobility and social aspects of rheumatic disorders). Thesis 1984.
111. Meyboom-de Jong B. Bejaarde patiënten; een onderzoek in twaalf huisartspraktijken (Elderly patients: a survey among twelve general practices). (Thesis) Groningen University. Meditekst, Lelystad 1989.
112. Huiskes CJA, Kraaimaat FW, Bijlsma JWJ, Schreurs PJG. De samenhang tussen lichamelijke en psychologische aspekten van de gezondheidsbeleving bij patiënten met reumatoïde artritis (Correlation between physical and psychological aspects of health perception among patients with rheumatoid arthritis). Tijdschr Soc Gezondh 1987; 65: 747.
113. Tilburg TG van, Verkregen en gewenste ondersteuning in het licht van eenzaamheids-ervaringen (Provision of and requirement of support in the light of perceived loneliness). (Thesis) Free University of Amsterdam, 1988.
114. Yoshino S, Uchida S. Sexual problems of women with rheumatoid arthritis. Arch Phys Med Rehab 1981; 62: 122-123.

115. Elst P, Sybesma T, Stad RJ van der, Prins APA, Hissink Muller W, Butter A den. Sexual problems in rheumatoid arthritis and ankylosing spondylitis. Arhritis Rheum 1984; 27: 217-220.
116. Central Bureau of Statistics. Industrial insurance board diagnosis statistics 1987 and statistical information supplied on request. 26 Nov. 1990.
117. Joint Medical Service. Statistical information 1988, Amsterdam 1989 and statistical information supplied on request, 9 July 1990.
118. Fries JF, Spitz P, Kraines RG, Holman HR. Measurement of patient outcome in arthritis. Arthritis Rheum 1980; 23: 137- 145.
119. Bradley LA. Psychosocial factors and disease outcomes in rheumatoid arthritis: old problems, new solutions, and a future agenda. Arthritis Rheum 1989; 32: 1611-1614.
120. Anderson KO, Bradley LA, Young LD, McDaniel LK, Wise CM. Rheumatoid arthritis: review of psychological factors related to etiology, effects, and treatment. Psychol Bull 1985; 98: 358-387.
121. Meenan RF, Gertman PM, Mason JH. Measuring health status in arthritis: the Arthritis Impact Measurement Scales. Arthritis Rheum 1980; 23: 146-152.
122. McFarlane AC, Brooks PM. An analysis of the relationship between psychological morbidity and disease activity in rheumatoid arthritis. J Rheumatol 1988; 15: 926-931.
123. McFarlane AC, Brooks PM. Determinants of disability in rheumatoid arthritis. Br J Rheumatol 1988; 27: 7-14.
124. Kraaimaat FW. Personally obtained information, 1991.
125. Sherrer YS, Bloch DA, Mitchell DM, Young DY, Fries JF. The development of disability in rheumatoid arthritis. Arthritis Rheum 1986; 29: 494-500.
126. Meenan RF, Kazis LE, Anderson JJ. The stability of health status in rheumatoid arthritis: a five-year study of patients with established disease. Am J Public Health 1988; 78: 1484- 1487.
127. Pincus T, Callahan LF, Sale WG, Brooks AL, Payne LE, Vaughn WK. Severe functional declines, work disability, and increased mortality in seventy-five rheumatoid arthritis patients studied over nine years. Arthritis Rheum 1984; 27:864-872.
128. Huiskes CJAE, Kraaimaat FW, Bijlsma JWJ. De ontwikkeling van de IRGL, een instrument om de gezondheid te meten bij patiënten met reuma (The development of thc IRGL, an instrument for measuring the health of patients with rheumatoid arthritis). Gedrag Gezondh 1990; 18: 78-89.

129. Jacoby RK, Jayson MIV, Cosh JA. Onset, early stages and prognosis of rheumatoid arthritis: a clinical study of 100 patients with 11-year follow-up. Br Med J 1973; 1: 96-100.
130. Hagglund KJ, Haley WE, Reveille JD, Alarcón GS. Predicting individual differences in pain and functional impairment among patients with rheumatoid arthritis. Arthritis Rheum 1989; 32: 851-858.
131. Brown GK, Nicassio PM. Development of a questionnaire for the assessment of active and passive coping strategies in chronic pain patients. Pain 1987; 31: 53-64.
132. Parker J, McRae C, Smarr K, Beck N, Frank R, Anderson S, Walker S. Coping strategies in rheumatoid arthritis. J Rheuma- tol 1988; 15: 1376-1383.
133. Blalock SJ, McEvoy deVellis B, deVellis RF, Sauter SH van. Self--evaluation processes and adjustment to rheumatoid arthritis. Arthritis Rheum 1988; 31: 1245-1251.
134. Frank RG, Beck NC, Parker JC, Kashani JH, Elliott TR, Haut AE, Smith E, Atwood C, Brownlee-Duffeck M, Kay DR. Depression in rheumatoid arthritis. J Rheumatol 1988; 15: 920-925.
135. Kraaimaat FW, Huiskes CJA. Stress en pijn bij patiënten met rheumatoïde arthritis (Stress and pain among patients with rheumatoid arthritis). Gedragstherapie 1989; 22: 267-277.
136. Sonderen E van. Measurement of social network and social support. Empirical results in relation to the Euridiss Instruments. Int J Health Sciences 1990; 1: 217-228.
137. Boer AH de. Leefsituatie en sociale steun bij chronisch zieken in vergelijking met gezonden; een secundaire analyse (Life situation and social support among the chronically ill compared with the healthy: a secondary analysis). National Institute for Health and Environmental Protection. Report no. 528904003, Bilthoven 1990.
138. Oberai B, Kirwan JR. Psychological factors in patients with chronic rheumatoid arthritis; Review. Ann Rheum Dis 1988; 47: 969-971.
139. Bradley LA, Young LD, Anderson KO, McDaniel LK, Turner RA, Agudelo CA. Psychological approaches to the management of arthritis pain. 1984; 19: 1353-1360.
140. Nicassio PM, Wallston KA, Callahan LF, Herbert M, Pincus T. The measurement of helplessness in rheumatoid arthritis. The development of the Arthritis Helplessness Index. J Rheumatol 1985; 12: 462-467.
141. Mazzuca SA. Does patient education in chronic disease have therapeutic value? J Chron Dis 1982; 35: 521-529.

142. Schiltmans MMC, Evers GCM. Zelfzorgvermogen en sociale ondersteuning bij reumapatiënten (Self-care capacity and social support among rheumatoid arthritis patients). Verpleegkunde 1989; 4: 195-200.
143. Lorig K, Konkel L, Gonzalez V. Arthritis patient education: a review of the literature. Patient Education Counseling 1987; 10; 207-252.
144. Taal E, Seydel E, Riemsma R, Brus H, Rasker JJ. Group education for patients with rheumatoid arthritis. Clin Rheumatol 1990; 9: 5-6.
145. Richardson MUS, Huiskes CJAE, Kraaimaat FW, Bijlsma JWJ. Outcome of group education aimed at coping with physical and psychological aspects of chronic rheumatoid arthritis. Clin Rheumatol 1990; 9: 9.
146. Riemsma R, Seydel E, Taal E, Brus H, Rasker JJ. Individual education to people with rheumatoid arthritis. Clin Rheumatol 1990; 9: 4-5.
147. Netherlands Federations of Associations of Patients with rheumatic disorders. Vooroordelen over reuma en de antwoorden daarop (Prejudices towards rheumatoid arthritis and appropriate responses). Brochure.
148. Turk DC. Factors influencing the adaptive process with chronic illness; Implications for intervention. In: Sarason IG, Spielberger CD (eds). Stress and anxiety. Volume 6. John Wiley & Sons, New York 1979.
149. Central Bureau of Statistics. Gezondheidsenquête 1989 (Health Interview Survey 1989). Quantitative informatie supplied on request. Voorburg/Heerlen.
150. Lamberts H. Morbidity in General Practice; Diagnosis related information from the monitoring project. Huisartsenpers B.V., Utrecht 1984.
151. Anonymous. Transition Project. Huisartsgeneeskunde University of Amsterdam. Quantitatieve informatie supplied on request. Amsterdam.
152. Nienhuis RLF. Verslag van een enquête naar het functioneren van een reumapolikliniek (Report on the functioning of a rheumatology clinic). Ned Tijdschr Geneeskd 1982; 126: 371-373.
153. Rijswijk MH van. Reumatologie en reumabestrijding. Een noodzaak! (Rheumatology and rheumatology control - a necessity!) Address delivered on 30 September 1986 on the occasion of appointment as Extraordinary Professor Rheumatology at Groningen University.
154. Lightfoot RW. Treatment of reumatoid arthritis. In: Arthritis and allied conditions; A textbook of rheumatology. McCarty DJ. Lea and Febiger, Philadelphia 1985: 668-676.
155. National Rheumatology Fund. Information leaflet on medicinal drugs. Medical Information Series 1990.

156. Huiskes CJAE, Bijlsma JWJ. Mondig ziek zijn: Reuma (Ill but self-assertive: rheumatic disorders). Bohn, Scheltema & Holkema. Utrecht/-Antwerp, 1989: 58-64.
157. Leufkens HGM, Ruter EM, Laar MAFJ van der, Bakker A. Estimation of prevalence of rheumatoid arthritis using prescription data from pharmacy records. In: Leufkens HGM, Pharmacy records in pharmacoepidemiology: studies on antiinflammatory and antirheumatic drugs. (Thesis) Utrecht University 1990: 204-214.
158. Bruin C de. Reuma, functionele toestand en zorg (Rheumatoid arthritis, functional condition and care). Practical medical training report, Groningen University, 1990.
159. Janssen M. Werking, bijwerking en keuze van niet-steroïde anti-inflammatoire middelen (Effectiveness, side-effects and choice of non-steroid anti-inflammatory drugs). In: Nieuwe inzichten in de pathogenese en behandeling van reumatoïde artritis (New insights into the pathogenesis and treatment of rheumatoid arthritis). Boerhaave Committee for Post-graduate Training in Medicine. Leiden 1989.
160. Jacobs J. Keyserling JA, Britton M, Morgan GJ, Wilkenfield J, Hutchings HC. The total cost of care and the use of pharmaceuticals in the management of reumatoid arthritis: the medical program. J Clin Epidemiol 1988; 41: 215-223.
161. Blackwell B. Psych MRC. Drug therapy; patient compliance. The New Engl J Med 1973; (august 2): 249-252.
162. Deyo RA, Inui TS, Sullivan B. Noncompliance with arthritis drugs: magnitude, correlates, and clinical implications. J Rheumatol 1981; 8: 931-936.
163. Inui TS, Carter WB, Pecoraro RE, Pearlman RA, Dohan JJ. Variations in patient compliance with common long-term drugs. Med Care 1980; 18: 986-993.
164. Bijlsma JWJ, Berge Henegouwen GP van, Boer SY de, Dijkmans BAC, Festen HPM, Janssen M. Preventie van gastroduodenale afwijkingen bij gebruik van niet-steroïde anti-inflammatoire geneesmiddelen (Prevention of gastroduodenal disorders from the use of non-steroid anti-inflammatory drugs). Ned Tijdschr Geneeskd 1991; 135: 45-48.
165. Gibson T, Clark B. Use of simple analgesics in rheumatoid arthritis. Ann Rheum Dis 1985; 44: 27-29.
166. Netherlands Association of General Practitioners. Suggesties voor beleid inzake reumabestrijding (Policy suggestions in respect of rheumatism control). Letter to the State Secretary of Health. Utrecht 26 september 1985.

167. Voorn TB. Chronische Ziekten in de huisartspraktijk (Chronic diseases in general practice). Wetenschappelijke Uitgeverij Bunge, Utrecht 1983.
168. Huiskes CJAE, Bijlsma JWJ. Mondig ziek zijn: Reuma (Ill but self-assertive: rheumatic disorders). Bohn, Scheltema & Holkema. Utrecht/-Antwerp, 1989: 65-69.
169. Buyten NT, Hoogen R van der, Monteny AE, in 't Veld HO, Lamberts H. Fysiotherapie: vierde in eerstelijns kwartet (Physiotherapy: fourth in primary-care quartet). Ned Tijdschr Fysiotherapie 1977; 11:374-380.
170. Central Bureau of Statistics. Statistical Yearbook 1990. SDU-uitgeverij, CBS-publications. The Hague 1990.
171. Brekel EJG van den. Fysiotherapie 1986/1988; Gezondheidsenquêtes (Physiotherapy 1986/1988; Health Interview Surveys). Mndber Gezondheid (CBS); 1989: (8) 13-17.
172. Weekers AMCL, Jonkers LV, Mostert HA, Pruyn JFA. Reuma; de aandoening en gevolgen, de wijkverpleegkundige zorgverlening en het beleid (Rheumatism: the disorder and consequences, district nursing care and policy). Institute for Socio-Scientific Research, Catholic University of Brabant. Tilburg, October 1989.
173. Twente Home Nursing Association. Reuma onderzoek Twente; de zorg vanuit het kruiswerk aan patiënten met RA (Rheumatism research in Twente; home-nursing care for RA patients). Bunnik National Home-Nursing Association 1988.
174. Sorber-Broekhuis H, Verstegen D, Vrijlandt M. Lastige patiënten worden gemaakt (Awkward patients are made). Publication for the theme-year. South-Holland Home Nursing Association, Zoetermeer 1990.
175. National Association of Social Workers. Beroepsprofiel van de maatschappelijk werker (Occupational profile of the social worker). Utrecht 1987.
176. Sonsbeek JLA van. Het raadplegen van alternatieve genezers in 1979 en 1981 (The consultation of alternative healers in 1979 and 1981). Mndber Gezondheid (CBS) 1983: (2) 5-15.
177. Riet G ter, Kleijnen J, Knipschild P. Acupunctuur en RA. De effectiviteit van acupunctuur (Acupuncture and RA. The effectiveness of acupuncture). Huisarts en Wetenschap 1989; 32(6): 228-229.
178. Jacobs JWG, Rasker JJ, Riel PLCM van, Gribnau FWJ, Putte LBA. Alternatieve behandelingswijzen bij reumatische aandoeningen; een literatuuronderzoek (Alternative forms of treatment for rheumatic disorders). Ned Tijdschr Geneeskd 1991; 135: 317- 322.

179. Visser GJ. Reuma en alternatieve geneeswijzen (Rheumatism and alternative forms of medicine). Conventional and alternative healers cooperation project; study no. 3. NIVEL, Utrecht 1989.
180. Commissie voor Reuma-onderzoek TNO. Naar een nieuw tijdsgewricht. Een strategische verkenning van de jaren negentig (TNO Committee for Rheumatology Research. Towards a new Juncture. A Strategic Survey of the 1990s.) Netherlands Institute for Preventive Health Care TNO, Leiden, 1990.
181. Korst JK van der, Meegdes JG. Reumazorg; zorgvuldige planning noodzakelijk (Rheumatism care: careful planning vital). Medisch Contact 1988; 43: 497-499.
182. Nationaal Ziekenhuisinstituut. Reumatologie in algemene, academische en categorale ziekenhuizen (Rheumatology in general, teaching and specialized hospitals). Utrecht, 1991.
183. Janssens MBJA. Landelijke Coördinatie Reumaresearch. De Standaard Diagnose Registratie van Reumatische Ziekten en Standaardisatie van de Reumaserologie (The Standard Diagnosis Registration of Rheumatic Diseases and Standardization of the Rheumatoid Factor). (Thesis) Erasmus University Rotterdam 1987.
184. Standard Diagnosis Registration. Quantitative information supplied on request. NIPG-TNO, Leiden 1991.
185. Jan van Breemen Instituut. Quantitative information supplied on request. Amsterdam 1989.
186. Leiden University Hospital. Quantitative information supplied on request. Leiden 1988.
187. Wijkel D. Ergotherapie als nazorg thuis; een pilot-study (Ergotherapy as after-care at home: a pilot study). Medisch Contact 1990; 45: 293-296.
188. Anonymous. Onderzoek naar ergotherapie in de eerste lijn; je bespaart er meer mee dan je uitgeeft (Research into ergotherapy in primary health care; the savings exceed the costs). In Beweging 1989; februari: 6-7.
189. Health Care Information Centre. National Medical Recording System (hospital admissions and nursing days). Annual reports and quantitative information supplied on request.
190. Health Care Information Centre. Ziekten in beeld. Informatie over verleende medische zorg bij een aantal ziektebeelden. Reumatoïde artritis (Diseases in Focus. Information on the Medical Care provided in respect of various clinical pictures. Rheumatoid arthritis. Utrecht 1990.
191. Dr. Daniël den Hoed Kliniek. 1989 Annual Report. Rotterdam, 1990.

192. "Sole Mio" Rheumatology Clinic. 1989 Socio-financial annual report and quantitative information supplied on request. 3 May 1991.
193. Meegdes JG. Reumatologie in beeld. Feiten en cijfers over de situatie van de reumatologie in Nederland en een blik naar de toekomst (Rheumatology in focus. Facts and figures on the rheumatology situation in the Netherlands and a glance at the future). National Hospitals Institute, Utrecht, 1988; no. 88.551.
194. Health Care Information Centre. Revalidatie Informatie Systeem (Rehabilitation Information System). Statistical information supplied on request. Utrecht.
195. Health Care Information Centre. Verpleeghuis Informatie Systeem (Nursing Home Information System). Annual reports and statistical information supplied on request. Utrecht.
196. Beighton P, Solomon L, Valkenburg HA. Rheumatoid arthritis in a rural South African Negro population. Ann Rheum Dis 1975; 34:136-141.
197. Henrard JC, Bennett PH, Burch RA. Rheumatoid arthritis in the Pima Indians of Arizona: An assessment of the clinical components of the New York criteria. Int J Epidemiol 1975; 4: 119-126.
198. Harvey J. Lotze M, Stevens MB, Lambert G, Jacobson D. Rheumatoid arthritis in a Chippewa band. Arthritis Rheum 1981; 24: 717-721.
199. Laine VAI. Rheumatic complaints in an urban population in Finland. Acta Rheum Scand 1962; 8: 81-88.
200. Behrend T, Lawrence JS, Behrend H, Fischer K. Prevalence of rheumatoid arthritis in rural Germany. Int J Epidemiol 1972; 1: 153-156.
201. O'Sullivan JB, Cathcart ES, Bolzan JA. Diagnostic criteria and the incidence of rheumatoid arthritis in Sudbury, Massachusetts. In: Bennett PH, Wood PHN (eds). Population studies of the rheumatic disease. Excerpta Medica Foundation, Amsterdam, 1968.
202. Euridiss. European research on incapacitating diseases and social support. Int J Health Sciences 1990; 1: 217-228.
203. Kazis LE, Meenan RF, Anderson JJ. Pain in the rheumatic diseases. Arthritis Rheum 1983; 26: 1017-1022.
204. Skevington SM. Psychological aspects of pain in rheumatoid arthritis: a review. Soc Sci Med 1986; 23: 567-575.
205. Liang MH, Rogers M, Larson M, Eaton HM, Murawski BJ, Taylor JE, Swafford J, Schur PH. The psychosocial impact of systemic lupus erythematosus and rheumatoid arthritis. Arthritis Rheum 1984; 27: 13-17.
206. Zaphiropoulos G, Burry HC. Depression in rheumatoid disease. Ann Rheum Dis 1974; 33: 132-135.

207. Fitzpatrick R, Newman S, Lamb R, Shipley M. Helplessness and control in rheumatoid arthritis. Int J Health Sciences 1990; 1: 17-23.
208. Ploeg FAE van der. De psychologische aspecten van reumatoïde artritis (The psychological aspects of rheumatoid arthritis). (Thesis) Groningen University, 1980.
209. Earle JR, Perricone PJ, Maultsby DM, Perricone N, Turner RA, Davis J. Psychosocial adjustment of rheumatoid arthritis patients from two alternative treatment settings. J Rheumatol 1979; 6: 80-87.
210. Fitzpatrick R, Newman S, Lamb R, Shipley M. Social relationships and psychological well-being in rheumatoid arthritis. Soc Sci Med 1988; 27: 399-403.
211. Vignos PJ. A comprehensive case and psychological factors in rehabilitation in chronic rheumatoid arthritis - a controlled study. J Chron Dis 1972; 24: 457-467.
212. Meenan RF, Yelin EH, Nevitt M, Epstein WV. The impact of chronic disease. A sociomedical profile of rheumatoid arthritis. Arhtritis Rheum 1981; 24: 544-549.
213. Yelin EH, Meenan RT, Nevit M. Work disability in rheumatoid arthritis: a relative impact of disease, social, and work factors. Ann Intern Med 1980; 93: 551-556.
214. Pincus T, Mitchell JM, Burkhauser RV. Substantial work disability and earnings losses in individuals less than age 65 with osteoarthritis: comparisions with rheumatoid arthritis. J Clin Epidemiol 1989; 42: 449-457.
215. Silman AJ. Are there secular trends in the occurrence and severity of rheumatoid arthritis? Scand J Rheumatology 1989; Suppl 79:25-30.
216. Lawrencre JS. Rheumatism in populations. London, Heinmann, 1977.
217. Silman AJ, Davies P, Evans SJW, Currey HLF. Is rheumatoid arthritis becoming less severe? J Chron Dis 1983; 36: 891-894.
218. Silman AJ. Recent trends in rheumatoid arthritis. Brit J Rheumatol 1986; 25: 328-330.
219. Silman AJ. Has the incidence of rheumatoid arthritis declined in the United Kingom? Brit J Rheumatol 1988; 27: 77-78.
220. Valkenburg HA. Rheumatoid arthritis, pregnancy and the pil - conflicting evidence. In: Rheumatology, current medical literature. Royal Society of Medicine, 1986; 5: 161-163.
221. Central Bureau of Statistics. Aandeel gezondheidszorg in het BNP (Share of health care in GNP). Information supplied on request 1990.
222. Swinkels H. Trendcijfers Gezondheidsenquête 1981-1988 (Health Interview Survey 1981-1988 trend figures). Mndber Gezondheid (CBS) 89: (9) 5-24.

223. Mos JM de. Oud en jong en de gezondheidszorg (Old and young and health care). Medisch Contact 1987; 42: 1402-1406.

Chapter 3

1. Harris, Jr. ED. Pathophysiology and implications for therapy. N. Engl. J. Med. 1990; 322: 1277-1289.

Chapter 4

1. Epidemiologisch Preventief Onderzoek Zoetermeer (EPOZ) (Zoetermeer Epidemiological Preventive Survey), fifth progress report, Volume 4, "Rheumatic Diseases". Erasmus University Rotterdam, Institute of Epidemiology, 1979.
2. Continue Morbiditeits Registratie Nijmeegs Universitair Huisartsen Instituut (Continuous Morbidity Surveillance Project, Nijmegen University General Practitioners Institute), 1985-1988. Data supplied on request.
3. Steering Committee on Future Health Scenarios. Chronische ziekten in het jaar 2005. Deel 1, Scenario's over diabetes mellitus 1990-2005. (Chronic Diseases in the year 2005. Volume 1, Scenarios on Diabetes Mellitus), Bohn, Scheltema & Holkema, Utrecht/Antwerp, 1990.
4. Cruijsen, H. Bevolkingsprognose 1989: meer buitenlandse migratie. (Population forecast 1989: more foreign migration). Mnd. Stat. Bevolk. 1990; 1: 6-38.
5. Harris, Jr. ED. Pathophysiology and implications for therapy. N. Engl. J. Med. 1990; 322: 1277-1289.
6. Rasker, J.J. Reuma hebben, wat betekent het RA-patient te zijn. (Rheumatic disease: What does it mean to be an RA-patient.) Lederle Nederland BV, Etten-Leur, 1984.
7. Witte, L.P. de, Tilli, D.J.P., Ticheler, A.J.G., Winants, B.A.C., Horst, F.G. van der, Linder, Sj. van der. Leven met een reumatische aandoening; een onderzoek naar de ervaren kwaliteit van leven bij 372 mensen met een reumatische aandoening (Living with a rheumatic disease: a study of the quality of life experienced by 372 persons with a rheumatic disease.) Instituut voor Revalidatie Vraagstukken (Institute for Rheumatic Problems), Hoensbroek 1989.

8. Draft Discussion Document on Health Policy. Purposive change for the years 1990-1995. Ministry of Welfare, Health and Cultural Affairs, Rijswijk, 1989.
9. Rheumatic Diseases Policy Document, Ministry of Welfare, Health and Cultural Affairs. Parliamentary Proceedings, Lower House, 1988-1989 session, 21010 no. 2, Rijswijk, 1989.
10. TNO Committee for Rheumatology Research. Naar een nieuw tijdsgewricht. Een strategische verkenning van de jaren negentig (Towards a new juncture. A strategic exploration of the nineteen nineties). TNO Institute of Preventive Health Care, Leiden, 1990.
11. Breedveld, F.C. Immuunmodulatie van reumatoïde artritis (Immunomodulation of rheumatoid arthritis). In: Nieuwe inzichten in de pathogenese en behandeling van reumatoïde artritis (New insights into the pathogenesis and treatment of rheumatoid arthritis). Boerhaave Commissie voor Postacademisch Onderwijs in de Geneeskunde (Boerhaave Committee for Postgraduate Education in Medicine), 1989: 115-121.
12. Hospital Facilities Council. Notitie ontwikkeling functie orthopedie (Memorandum: development of the function of orthopaedics). CvZ (Hospital Facilities Council) no. 4621-90, Utrecht, 1991.

Chapter 5

1. Hospital Facilities Council. Notitie ontwikkeling functie orthopedie (Memorandum: development of the function of orthopaedics). CvZ (Hospital Facilities Council) no. 4621-90, Utrecht, 1991.
2. Science Policy Advisory Council (RAWB). Prioriteiten in het Gezondheidsonderzoek (Priorities in Health Research). Government Publication Distribution Centre, The Hague, 1983.
3. Gezondheidsraad (Health Council). Jaarboek 1985 (Yearbook 1985), Gezondheidsraad, The Hague, 1985.
4. Stimuleringsprogramma Gezondheidsonderzoek (SGO) (Health Research Promotion Programme). Parliamentary Proceedings, Lower House, 1985-1986 session, no. 19363, Rijswijk, 1986.
5. Rheumatic Diseases Policy Document. Ministry of Welfare, Health and Cultural Affairs. Dutch Lower House, 1988-1989 session, 21010 no. 2, Rijswijk, 1989.
6. Chronic Diseases Policy Memorandum. The chronically ill on the sidelines. Ministry of Welfare, Health and Cultural Affairs. Parliamen-

tary Proceedings, Lower House, 1990-1991 session, 22025, no. 1, Rijswijk, 1991.

7. Health Policy Document. Ministry of Welfare, Health and Cultural Affairs. Rijswijk, in preparation.
8. TNO Committee for Rheumatology Research. Naar een nieuw tijdsgewricht. Een strategische verkenning van de jaren negentig (Towards a new juncture. A strategic exploration of the nineteen nineties). TNO Institute of Preventive Health Care, Leiden, 1990.
9. Bos, G.A.M. van den. Zorgen van en voor chronisch zieken (Worries of and caring for the chronically ill). Ph.D. thesis. Universiteit van Amsterdam, 1989.

APPENDIX

DIAGNOSIS AND TREATMENT OF RHEUMATOID ARTHRITIS

Prof. M.H. van Rijswijk, Prof. J.J. Rasker

1. Introduction

This appendix describes the diagnostic and therapeutic possibilities with respect to rheumatoid arthritis (RA). This is preceded by brief descriptions of the clinical picture and of a typical RA-patient. Finally, a number of future expectations and targets are presented.

2. The clinical picture of rheumatoid arthritis

RA is one of the most serious rheumatic diseases. The disease is characterized by chronic inflammation of multiple joints (polyarthritis). Although there is a certain predilection for the small joints of the hands and forefeet, the inflammation can manifest itself in virtually any joint. The cause of RA has not yet been discovered. The chronic joint inflammation is probably caused by a continuous reaction by T-cells (the cells of the body's defence mechanism) which turn against endogenous constituents. It seems reasonable to assume that such a reaction can be set in motion by antigen structures in micro-organisms which display correspondences with endogenous antigens occurring mainly in the joints. Normally such a reaction will be suppressed by the defence system's regulatory mechanisms. Failure of this regulatory mechanism can lead to chronic joint inflammation.

This inflammation of the joints is the fundamental characteristic of RA, and leads to pain, stiffness, function impairment and breakdown of cartilage, bone and sockets. Although attention focuses strongly on joint deformity when considering RA, it should be borne in mind that this is in fact a systemic disease, which affects the whole body and in which anaemia, tiredness and muscle breakdown all contribute to the ultimate degree of the patient's handicap. The enormous limitations which a patient with RA can experience in carrying out even the most basic activities can lead to severe disruption of daily life. The result is a substantial reduction in self-reliance and an increase in dependence.

3. Brief description of a typical patient

A woman in her 32nd year, a few weeks after the birth of her second child, develops problems in the joints of her hands, wrists and forefeet. She suffers severe morning stiffness and is no longer able to place her child in the bath. She is also extremely tired. Although treatment with painkillers such as Indomethacin and therapeutic drugs such as Hydroxy-chloroquin and, later, gold injections, each produce some improvement, after each treatment the disease eventually reappears. More and more joints are affected, and the woman is forced to give up her part-time secretarial job.

Because she develops extremely painful hammer-toes, with hard skin and pressure points on the soles of her feet, she is given orthopaedic shoes. She finds these appalling at first, though they do enable her to walk with less pain. She also develops nodules on her elbows, and her hip starts to become so painful that she has to use a wheelchair for a time. Thanks to an artificial hip implanted by an orthopaedic surgeon, followed a few years later by an artificial knee, she is once again able to walk independently and is no longer completely dependent on others.

The patient is now 55 years old and has moved to a smaller, modified dwelling. Her husband has had to give up his career because he has to care for her in the mornings and the evenings. Each year they holiday in Groot Stokkert, the holiday centre run by the National Rheumatism Fund. This gives them great enjoyment, since he can go on walks and she is able to swim in the warm pool.

4. Diagnostic possibilities

The diagnosis rheumatoid arthritis is established on the basis of a combination of patient records, physical examination, laboratory tests and the results of X-ray examination. Good clinical skills are a precondition for establishing the diagnosis RA at the earliest possible stage of the disease, i.e. when joint damage is still limited or absent. In the first place this demands experience in observing the symptoms of arthritis; in the second place, expert experience is needed in order to distinguish RA from other forms of polyarthritis. This is of great importance for the initiation of correct treatment.

Laboratory tests can provide information to supplement patient records and physical examination. A positive rheumatoid factor test in a person with arthritis is a strong argument for an RA diagnosis. Selectivity is needed, however, in seeking such a diagnosis in the case of general symptoms affecting the postural and locomotory system. If the person concerned does not have arthritis, then he or she does not have RA, whatever the result of the rheumatoid factor test. It can be assumed in advance that there is at least a 5% probability of a positive result without any disease being present. A negative result is also of limited value, since in a patient in the early stages of RA the rheumatoid factor test can (still) prove negative. General biochemical indicators (e.g. blood sedimentation) can give an impression of the activity and extent of the disease. For diagnosis, however, it should be borne in mind that, particularly where the arthritis is limited to small joints, the degree of blood sedimentation may not always be raised.

Specific expertise is also required for the radiological examination: the more subtle abnormalities which can be present in the early stages are easily missed. For early diagnosis of RA, joint discussion of the X-rays by the clinician and the X-ray diagnostician is essential. In selected cases, it may be useful to supplement the information using more sophisticated image-forming techniques (scintigraphy, MRI).

5. Therapeutic possibilities

A great deal has changed for the RA-patient in recent decades, in spite of the absence of any fundamental breakthroughs. Better drug therapy and surgical therapy mean that there are now few patients who become so severely disabled that they are condemned to a wheelchair. And yet RA is and remains one of the most serious rheumatological disorders, whose consequences for the patient are often greatly underestimated. As total cure of the disease is not (yet) possible, control of the consequences and optimization of the daily functioning of the patient occupy an extremely important position in the RA-care picture.

For a proper understanding of the total range of measures which are needed for the treatment and support of patients with this disease, it is necessary to bear in mind that joint damage is an irreversible, cumulative process. Once damaged, a joint is subject to greatly accelerated wear (secondary arthrosis).

A brief description is given below of the therapeutic possibilities with respect to RA, classified according to the type of therapy: drug therapy, non-drug therapy and surgical therapy.

a. Drug therapy

The drugs used for treating RA can be divided into the non-steroid anti-inflammatory non-steroid agents (NSAIDs) and the slow-acting anti-rheumatic drugs, also referred to as "disease modifying anti-rheumatic drugs" (DMARDs). NSAIDs are used mainly to counteract the symptoms of joint inflammation and have no effect on the cause of the disease itself. DMARDs are used to suppress the activity of the disease itself as far as possible and have a favourable effect on its course.

NSAIDs

These drugs have a painkilling, fever-reducing and inflammation-inhibiting action. The latter effect is based on inhibition of the synthesis of prostaglandins, which play an important role in the inflammation process and are responsible among other things for pain and stiffness symptoms. Treatment with NSAIDs can produce a considerable reduction in these symptoms, thus increasing freedom of movement, which in turn means that exercise therapy can be more effective. In this way mobility restriction and loss of function can be controlled to an important degree.

DMARDs

The activity of the disease process itself can in many cases be noticeably reduced using these slow-acting, "disease modifying" anti-rheumatic drugs. Examples of these medications include anti-malaria agents, sulphasalazine, gold preparations, d-pencillamin and cytostatics. As a rule these drugs require several months to take effect. In extremely severe cases it can be useful to bridge this baseline period with corticosteroids. If the above agents have insufficient effect it is often still possible to bring the disease under control using immunosuppressive agents. A specific monitoring regime is associated with each of these agents in order to signal any side effects in good time.

Local injections

Where there is local activity of RA in one or more joints, while the disease is otherwise in a resting phase, local injections administered directly to the joint concerned can often bring about a substantial improvement without it being necessary to make any changes to the other drug therapy programme. Intra-articular treatment such as this may involve the administering of anti-inflammatory agents, particularly in the form of locally-acting corticosteroids, or of a drug-based "synovectomy", in which the inflamed synovial membrane is removed as far as possible using chemical or radioactive substances.

b. Non-drug therapy

Rest
Dosed rest still forms an important part of the treatment, especially during active phases of the disease. Rest may be prescribed in the form of bed-rest and/or the use of immobilization splints. The favourable results achieved through dosed rest include a reduction in inflammatory activity, relief from pain and limitation of joint damage.

Physiotherapy
Physiotherapy, and in particular exercise therapy, is an essential part of the treatment of RA. Exercise therapy can be given in two forms: (1) passive, in order to retain mobility as far as possible and to prevent joints "setting'; (2) active, geared primarily to improving freedom of movement and strengthening the muscles; the latter is important for the stability of the joints.

Application of warmth/cold is important, since this can produce a temporary reduction in pain and stiffness, resulting in greater effectiveness of the exercise therapy. An additional advantage of physiotherapy lies in the attention given to the patient and to the disease. This has a positive effect on the patient's ability to come to terms with and accept the disease, and creates opportunities for further explanation (for example about a regimen for living). The effectiveness of the treatment can be increased still further by giving exercise therapy in warm water (hydrotherapy).

Ergotherapy
Ergotherapists play an important role in achieving measures geared towards the various forms of adaptation. The term "adaptation" requires some explanation. In the first place this term refers to the use of appliances which enable the patient to cope with an unadapted environment. The use of handgrips to enable a patient to turn an

ordinary key in a lock and turn an ordinary tap on and off is an example of such an appliance. In this way the patient adapts to his or her environment. However, if a modified tap or electrical door-opener is fitted, then the immediate environment has adapted to the patient. A final possibility is a more general adaptation of the environment, for example in the sense of the accessibility of public buildings.

A slightly different approach to the term "adaptation" is the adaptation of the patient to the disease, for example through ergonomic instruction, learning alternative techniques which enable a number of essential daily actions to be performed, such as sitting, lying, getting out of a chair, draining a pan of potatoes, tying a knot, putting on socks, etc. An important aspect of the ergonomic instruction is that the patients learn the techniques for performing daily activities in such a way that the joints are not unnecessarily or incorrectly loaded. This aspect can be summarized using the term "joint-protecting measures". Work adaptation, retraining, transport facilities and adapted recreation facilities should also be mentioned here.

c. Rheumatoid surgery

Rheumatoid surgery can be divided into two groups:

1. Preventive surgery, particularly in the form of synovectomy, in which the inflamed membrane covering the joint (the synovial membrane) is removed as far as possible with the aim of preventing further damage to the joints and tendons. This form of surgery is often used for hands and wrists.
2. Reconstructive surgery, such as the repair of damaged tendons, the implantation of artificial joints in hands and, of course, the larger joint replacement operations such as knee and hip replacements.

In former years arthrodesis (setting of a joint) was the only possibility when a joint had become totally damaged as a result of the chronic inflammation process.

At the end of the 1960s the hip arthroplasty (artificial hip) and later also knee arthroplasty (artificial knee) were introduced. These enabled many patients with a long history of RA to be helped successfully. The replacement of a damaged joint produces a reduction in pain and an improvement in function. Initially, due to the limited life of the artificial joints, only older patients were considered for these operations. Nowadays, however, the continuing improvements in both the prostheses and the surgical techniques makes it possible to operate on younger patients as well. It is now also possible to replace prostheses.

6. Future expectations and targets

Fortunately, promising developments are taking place in the treatment of patients with RA. Both research into new drug therapy and surgical treatment methods and developments relating to the organization and coordination of care offer good prospects.

a. Drug therapy

NSAIDs
The majority of patients tolerate NSAIDs well, but some 10 to 20% suffer unacceptable side-effects (particularly stomach ulcers). Research into the possibilities of intervening more selectively in the process of prostaglandin synthesis is currently in full swing and will it is hoped lead to preparations becoming available which match the desired effects of the present generation of NSAIDs, but without the undesirable side-effects. The synthetic prostaglandin-analogues which have now become available offer the possibility of counteracting the undesirable effects on the mucous membrane of the stomach. It is likely that it will soon also be possible to synthesize inflammation-inhibiting prostaglandins.

DMARDs
There is currently a very clear trend in the drug-based treatment of RA away from the gradually increasing regime which was formerly the norm (whereby more powerful drugs were gradually prescribed) towards a treatment strategy in which the drug-based intervention follows the regime outlined below:
- start of treatment at an early stage;
- selection of "quick"-acting drugs;
- choice of agents with proven effectiveness.

This intensification is aimed at preventing further joint damage. In the majority of patients with RA considerable damage to the joints arises within as little as two years of the onset of the disease. Once it has occurred, damage cannot be undone, and a joint once damaged is subject to greatly accelerated wear (secondary arthrosis). Examples of agents which have recently come into favour include azathioprine, salazopyrine and methotrexate. Under the new strategy treatment using cytostatics can begin within only a few months, something which in the classic treatment regime generally occurred only after several years.

T-cell manipulation

In addition to the agents which are directed at a more general suppression of the undesirable reaction of the defence system, such as cytostatics, other, more specific methods are being developed to suppress precisely those T-cells which are responsible for sustaining the inflammation of the joint. This might be attained by isolation and selective cultures of these T-cells. With the aid of these T-cells or constituents thereof, a targeted defence reaction can then be stimulated in the patient (comparable with vaccination). On the basis of animal experiments and initial results with RA-patients, this appears to be a promising development.

Cytokins

Another recent development relates to the rapidly increasing knowledge on the role of cytokins. Important cytokins include interleukin 1, interleukin 6 and tumour-necrosis factor. Cytokins are small protein molecules which transfer the signals between the various cells involved in the inflammation process (comparable to hormones). They are largely responsible for sustaining an inflammation and for the resultant damage. With the help of DNA-technology, cytokins and their respective inhibitors can be created in the laboratory. Using products such as these it will be possible in the future to achieve effective suppression of the inflammation of the joints and to limit the damage.

b. Surgery

The developments in surgery involve improvements in existing prostheses and the development of new ones. The shoulder prosthesis is already regularly implanted and there are promising developments in the area of ankle and elbow prostheses. Through the setting up of special rheumatology teams and the organization of conferences, rheumatologists, orthopaedic and plastic surgeons, rehabilitation physicians, ergotherapists and physiotherapists attempt to coordinate their individual activities as far as possible. By a combination of optimization of indications and the timing of operations, and increasing quality of the post-operative treatment, the end-result for the patient is continually improving.

c. Coordination of care

Given the wide range of implications of RA for daily functioning, the complexity of the rules and bureaucracy involved in the implementation of social security regulations, lack of expert experience among the implementing organizations, and insufficient communication, the desired total package of measures is often difficult to achieve. Adequate case management performed on the basis of experience offers good prospects for achieving "customized" care. An important starting point is ensuring that everyone is communicating on the same wavelength; the deployment of specialized nursing personnel is of particular importance here.

Annex 1

A classification system for rheumatic diseases (1)

a. Polyarthritis of unknown origin, including rheumatoid arthritis, ankylosing spondylitis, Reiter's syndrome and arthitis with psoriaris;
b. The connective tissue diseases, including genralized lupus erythematosus, scleroderma, dermatomyositis, polymyositis and the vasculitis syndromes; rheumatoid arthritis and Sjögren's syndrome are generally counted among these;
c. Acute rheumatism and other forms of post-infectious arthritis;
d. Degenerative articular diseases: primary and secondary arthritis;
e. Non-articular rheumatism, including tendinitis, tendovaginitis and busitis;
f. Diseases often associated with arthritis, such as certain intestinal diseases, sarcoidosis and Henoch/Schönlein's purpura;
g. Infectious arthritis;
h. Traumatic and neurological disorders, including neuropathic arthropathy (Charcot's joints) and Sudeck arthropathy;
i. Rheumatic disorders resulting (possibly) from biochemical or endocrine disorders, such as gout, hyperparathyroid and acromegaly; these may also be taken as including chondrocalcinosis caused by pyrophosphate crystals. In the case of the latter diseases metabolic disorders are even present in the joints. Similarly metabolic disorders in the joint are assumed to be behind the onset of primary arthritis;
j. Benign and malignant neoplasms;
k. Hypersensitive reactions to certain allergens or drugs, including serum sickness and the lupus erythematosus syndrome caused by certain drugs;
l. Hereditary or congenital disorders;
m. Various other diseases, including synovitis villonodularis pigmentosa, Bechet's syndrome, erythema nodosum and aseptic bone necrosis.

(1) Cats A, Putte LBA van der. Reumatische ziekten (Rheumatic diseases). In: Interne Geneeskunde (Internal Medicine), Ottolander GJH den (ed.), Bohn, Scheltema & Holkema, Utrecht, 1989: 343.

Annex 2

ARA diagnostic criteria for rheumatoid arthritis (1)

The diagnosis of rheumatoid arthritis is made by utilizing a number of criteria. Depending on the presence and duration a distinction is drawn between:

a. *Classic rheumatoid arthritis*: the patient satisfies at least seven criteria.
b. *Definite rheumatoid arthritis*: the patient satisfies at least five criteria.
c. *Probable rheumatoid arthritis*: the patient satisfies at least three criteria.
d. *Possible rheumatoid arthritis*: the patient satisfies two criteria.
e. For the first three categories, at least one of criteria a through e must be continuously in evidence for at least six weeks. The diagnosis of "possible rheumatoid arthritis" requires a continuous period of at least three weeks.

Criteria

a. Morning stiffness of at least 15 minutes.
b. Pain on motion or tenderness in at least one joint (observed by a physician).
c. Swelling in at least one joint that represents soft tissue thickening or fluid (observed by a physician).
d. Swelling of at least one other joint, observed by a physician: an interval free of joint symptoms between the two joint involvements may not be more than three months.
e. Symmetrical joint swelling (i.e. simultaneous involvement of the same joint on both sides of the body) with simultaneous involvement of midphalangeal, metacarpophalangeal, or metatarsophalangeal joints is acceptable without absolute symmetry; terminal phalangeal joint involvement does not satisfy this criteria.
f. Subcutaneous nodules over bone prominences, on extensor surfaces or in juxta-articular regions (observed by a physician).
g. Radiographic changes typical of rheumatoid arthritis, which must include at least bony decalcification localized to or greatest around the involved joint and not just a degenerative changes. Degenerative changes do not exclude patients from any group classified as rheumatoid arthritis.

h. Positive agglutination test: demonstration of the "rheumatoid factor" by any method that has been negative in 95% or more of normal controls in two laboratories.
i. Poor mucin precipitate from synovial fluid.
j. Characteristic histologic changes in synovial membrane with three or more of the following: marked villous hypertrophy, proliferation of superficial synovial cells, marked infiltration of chronic inflammatory cells (lymphocytes or plasma cells predominating), with tendency to form "lymphoid nodules", deposition of compact fibrin, either on surface or interstitially, foci of necrosis.
k. Characteristic histologic changes in nodules showing granulomatous foci with central zones of cell necrosis, surrounded by a palisade of proliferated mononuclear cells, peripheral fibrosis and chronic inflammatory cell infiltration, largely perivascular.

Any of the following features will exclude a patient from all categories of rheumatoid arthritis.

Exclusions

a. The typical rash of systemic lupus erythematosus (with butterfly distribution, follicle plugging and areas of atrophy).
b. High concentration of LE cells (four or more in two smears prepared from heparinized blood incubated not over two hours).
c. Histologic evidence of periarteritis nodosa with segmental necrosis of arteries associated with nodular leukocytic infiltration extending perivascularly and tending to include many eosinophils.
d. Weakness of neck, trunk and pharyngeal muscles for persistent muscle swelling or dermatomyositis.
e. Definite scleroderma, not limited to the fingers.
f. A clinical picture characteristic of rheumatic fever with migratory joint involvement and evidence of endocarditis, especially if accompanied by subcutaneous nodules or erythema marginatum or chorea. (An elevated anti-streptolysin titer will not rule out the diagnosis of rheumatoid arthritis).
g. A clinical picture characteristic of gouty arthritis with acute attacks of swelling, redness, and pain, especially if relieved by colchicine.
h. Tophi.
i. A clinical picture characteristic of acute infectious arthritis of bacterial or viral origin with: an acute focus of infection or in close association with a disease of known infectious origin; chills; fever; an

acute joint involvement, usually migratory initially (especially if there are organisms in the joint fluid or there is a response to antibiotic therapy).

j. Tubercule bacilli in the joints or historic evidence of joint tuberculosis.

k. A clinical picture characteristic of Reiter's syndrome with urethritis and conjunctivitis associated with acute joint involvement, usually migratory initially.

l. A clinical picture characteristic of the shoulder-hand syndrome, with unilateral involvement of shoulder and hand and diffuse swelling of the hand followed by atrophy and contractures.

m. A Clinical picture characteristic of hypertrophic pulmonary osteoparthropathy with clubbing of fingers or hypertrophic periostitis along the shafts of the long bones, especially if an intrapulmonary lesion or other associated disease is present.

n. A clinical picture characteristic of neuroarthropathy, with condensation and destruction of bones of involved joints and with associated neurologic findings.

o. Homogentisic acid in the urine detectable grossly with alkalinization.

p. Histologic evidence of sarcoid or a positive Kveim test.

q. Multiple myeloma, as evidence by a marked increase in plasma cells in the bone marrow or Bence Jones protein in the urine.

r. Characteristic skin lesions of erythema nodosum.

s. Leukemia or lymphoma with characteristic cells in peripheral blood, bone marrow, or tissues.

t. Agammaglobulinemia.

(1) Derived from: Ropes MW, Bennett GA, Cobb S, Jacox R, Jessar Ra. Revision of diagnostic criteria for rheumatoid arthritis. Bull Rheum Dis 1958; 9:175-176.

Annex 3

New classification criteria for rheumatoid arthritis (1)

In 1987 the American Rheumatism Association (ARA) drew up new criteria for the classification of rheumatoid arthritis:

Criterion	Definition*
1. Morning stiffness	Morning stiffness in or around joints for at least one hour (up to maximum improvement);
2. Arthritis of three or more joints or joint-groups	Swelling in at least three joints or groups of joints that represent soft tissue thickening or fluid, not bony over growth (observed by a physician); the 14 possible localizations are: right or left PIP joints; MCP joints, wrist, elbow, knee, ankle and MTP joints;
3. Arthritis of hands or wrists	Swelling of at least one wrist, MCP or PIP joint;
4. Symmetrical arthritis	Simultaneous involvement of the same joint on both sides (no absolute symmetry required for PIP, MCP and MTP joints);
5. Rheumatoid nodules	Subcutaneous nodules over bone prominences, on extensive surfaces or in juxta-articular regions (observed by a physician);
6. Positive serological reaction for rheumatoid factor	Demonstration of the rheumatoid factor by any method that has been positive in not over 5% of normal controls;
7. Radiographic changes	Presence of characteristic X-ray features for rheumatoid arthritis of the hand and/or wrist (front-rear shots), consisting at least of erosions or clear peri-articular decalcification.

* Abbreviations:

PIP = proximal interphalangeal
MCP = metacarpophalangeal
MTP = metatarsophalangeal

Four of the seven criteria must be satisfied for classification as RA. Criteria 1-4 must have been present for at least six weeks. A distinction is no longer drawn between the various forms of RA (see Annex 2).

(1) Derived from: Arnett FC, Edworthy SM, Bloch DA. The American Rheumatism Association 1987 revised criteria for the classification of rheumatoid arthritis. Arthritis Rheum 1988; 31:315-324.

Annex 4

Rheumatoid arthritis and allied conditions according to the ICHPPC-2-defined (1)

Rheumatoid arthritis and allied conditions (714)
incl. ankylosing spondylitis
excl. psoriatic arthropathy (217, **6961**)
Inclusion in the rubric requires:

A. For rheumatoid arthritis - all of the following:

a. Presence or history of an episode of joint pain involving three or more limb joints which occur in groups (e.g. PIPs or MCPs on one side count only as a single joint);
b. Swelling, subluxation or ankylosis of at least three limb joints including one hand, wrist, or foot with symmetry of at least one joint pair (Joints excluded are hips, DIPs, fifth PIPs, firs CMCs and first MTPs);
c. X-ray features of grade 2, 3, or more of erosive arthritis in the hands, wrists, or feet;
d. Positive serological reaction for rheumatoid factor.

B. For ankylosing spondylitis:
Characteristic radiological appearance;
Consider: (288, **7194**) Pain in joint; (289, **7190**) Swelling of joint; (231, **725-**) Arthritis NYD of NOS.

* Abbreviations:
DIP = distal interphalangeal,
PIP = proximal interphalangeal,
CMC = carpometacarpal,
MTP = metatarsophalangeal.

(1) ICHPPC-2-defined. International Classification of Health Problems in Primary Care. Oxford, Oxford University Press, 1983.

Annex 5

Number of patients with rheumatoid arthritis in 2005 compared with 1990 according to the static model

Table 1 Number of patients with rheumatoid arthritis in the period 1990-2005 by age and sex on the basis of the prevalences in the EPOZ(1)

	1990		2005		Increase 1990-2005 absolute (%)			
	Men	Women	Men	Women	Men		Women	
20 - 44	10,497	4,237	10,755	3,726	258	(2.5)	- 511	(-12.1)
45 - 64	17,287	40,923	24,938	56,612	7,651	(44.3)	15,689	(38.3)
65 - 79	9,227	34,537	10,856	38,305	1,629	(17.7)	3,768	(10.9)
80+	1,617	20,449	2,129	27,216	512	(31.7)	6,767	(33.1)
Total	38,628	100,146	48,678	125,859	10,050	(26.0)	25,713	(25.7)

Table 2 Number of patients with rheumatoid arthritis (including ankylosing spondylitis) in the period 1990-2005 by age and sex on the basis of the prevalences in the NUHI (2)

	1990		2005		Increase 1990-2005 absolute (%)			
	Men	Women	Men	Women	Men		Women	
0 - 19	1,416	326	1,459	288	42	(3.0)	-38	(-11.7)
20 - 44	7,066	12,292	6,818	13,073	-248	(-3.5)	781	(6.4)
45 - 64	12,337	15,177	17,601	21,073	5,264	(42.7)	5,896	(38.8)
65 - 79	8,820	23,405	10,363	25,802	1,543	(17.5)	2,397	(10.2)
80+	2,879	9,815	3,719	12,992	840	(29.2)	3,177	(32.4)
Total	32,519	61,015	39,960	73,228	7,441	(22.9)	12,213	(20.0)

1. Zoetermeer Epidemiological Preventive Survey (EPOZ), 5th progress report, Volume 4, Rheumatic Diseases. Erasmus University Rotterdam, Institute of Epidemiology, 1979.
2. Continuous Morbidity Surveillance Project, Nijmegen University General Practitioners Institute, 1985-1988. Data supplied on request.

Annex 6

Description of a "typical" Dutch rheumatoid arthritis patient who was the subject of the questions in the Delphi questionnaire

Most of the questions in the Delphi study related to the entire group of RA-patients. In a number of cases, however, the questionnaire looked more closely at the problems of a specific RA-patient. As the manifestation of RA can vary considerably from patient to patient, not everyone will understand the same thing under terms such as "an average RA-patient". We therefore described a "typical" Dutch RA-patient, about whom a number of questions were formulated in the questionnaire.

The rheumatoid arthritis patient:
The patient is a female aged 40. The disease began insidiously. Subsequently she remembers that the first symptoms began a year previously. On diagnosis she is experiencing pain and swellings in the wrist and the joints of the fingers and toes. She is also troubled with generalized morning stiffness which lasts until approximately half an hour after she has got out of bed, combined with general malaise. One year after the establishment of the diagnosis there are subcutaneous nodules present on the extension side of the elbow. The rheumatoid factor is present, at a moderately high level.

Annex 7

Acknowledgements and composition of Delphi panel

We should like to express our thanks to the large number of experts who cooperated in the Delphi study:

Mrs. M. Belles, ergotherapist, Het Groene Kruis, Stadskanaal
Prof. F.C. Breedveld, rheumatologist, Leiden University Hospital
Prof. J.W.J. Bijlsma, rheumatologist, Utrecht University Hospital
Mrs. E.W.E. Draaier-Jansen, physician, GG & GD Utrecht and member of the administrative board of the National Rheumatism Fund, Zeist
Mrs. G.T.J. van Dijk-Bösecke, rheumatology nurse, Medisch Spectrum Twente, Enschede
Prof. J.C. van Es, emeritus professor of general practice, Chairman of the Health Research Promotion Programme, member of the Health Research Council, Amersfoort
Prof. T.E.W. Feltkamp, immunologist, Central Blood Transfusion Laboratory of the Dutch Red Cross, Amsterdam
Dr. H.S. Goei The, rheumatologist, "De Wever" Hospital, Heerlen
Mrs. K. Holwerda-Straver, rheumatology nurse, Groningen University Hospital
A.F. van Helmond, psychologist, St. Maarten's Clinic, Nijmegen
Prof. A.J.C. Huffstadt, emeritus professor of plastic and reconstructive surgery, State University of Groningen
Mrs. E.M. IJssennagger, area nurse for rheumatic diseases and rehabilitation, Twente Home Nursing Service, Hengelo
Mrs. J.J. Koning, member of the Netherlands Federation of Associations of Patients with Rheumatic Diseases, Egmond-Binnen
Prof. J.K. van det Korst, rheumatologist, Jan van Breemen Institute, Amsterdam
Prof. F.W. Kraaimaat, clinical psychologist, Utrecht University Hospital
Mrs. M.A.H. van Kuyk-Minis, ergotherapist, St. Maartenskliniek, Nijmegen
Prof. H. Lamberts, Institute of General Practice, University of Amsterdam
Prof. G.J. Lankhorst, rehabilitation physician, Free University Hospital, Amsterdam
H. van der Leeden, rheumatologist, Merwede Hospital, Dordrecht
Prof. A.J. van der Linden, orthopaedic surgeon, Maastricht University Hospital
Prof. Sj. van der Linden, rheumatologist, Maastricht University Hospital

Prof. B. Meyboom-de Jong, Institute of General Practice, State University of Groningen

H.A. Mostert, Nurse/nursing officer, Industrial Insurance Board of Interzorg Holland, Zoetermeer

Dr. R.L.F. Nienhuis, rheumatologist, Beatrixoord, Haren

F.G.J. Oosterveld, physiotherapist, Medisch Spectrum Twente, Enschede

J. van de Rest, Director, National Rheumatism Fund, The Hague

Mrs. E.B.W. Ros-Fuchs, social worker, St. Maartenskliniek, Nijmegen

Prof. P.M. Rozing, orthopaedic surgeon, Leiden University Hospital

H.J. Smid, Head of the Health Promotion and Disease Prevention Division, Ministry van Welfare, Health and Cultural Affairs, Rijswijk

Mrs. C.K. Smit, ergotherapist/policy officer, Jan van Breemen Institute, Amsterdam

Dr. P.H.M. Spauwen, plastic surgeon, Groningen University Hospital

R.F. Swens, consultant physician, Regional Health Insurance Council, Rijn/IJsselland, Doorwerth

S. Terpstra, economist, Long-term planning bureau, University Hospital Groningen

Prof. H.A. Valkenburg, emeritus professor of epidemiology, Director of the Institute of Non-hospital Medical Research, Free University of Amsterdam

Mrs. D. Verstegen, member of the Netherlands Federation of Associations of Patients with Rheumatic Diseases, The Hague

C. van Winzum, Medical Director, Merck Sharp en Dohme B.V., Haarlem

Our special thanks also go out to Prof. H.A. Valkenburg, emeritus professor of epidemiology, Institute for Non-hospital Medical Research, Free University of Amsterdam, Prof. F.W. Kraaimaat, clinical psychologist, Utrecht University Hospital, and R. Riemsma and E. Taal, both attached as psychologists to the Department of Psychology, Twente University of Technology, for their advice on the background study. We would also like to thank Dr. J.W.G. Jacobs, rheumatologist at the Department of Rheumatology, Utrecht University Hospital, for his advice regarding the whole report. We are grateful to Mrs. E. du Mosch for her secretarial support.

List of abbreviations

ADL	:	Activities of Daily Living
AMW	:	General Social Work
ARA	:	American Rheumatism Association
CBS	:	Central Bureau of Statistics
CNSLD	:	Chronic Non-Specific Lung Disease
CR-TNO	:	TNO Committee for Rheumatology Research
DMARD	:	Disease Modifying Anti-Rheumatic Drug
DSM	:	Diagnostic and Statistical Manual of Mental Disorders
EPOZ	:	Zoetermeer Epidemiological Preventive Survey
GAK	:	Industrial Insurance Administration Office
GMD	:	Joint Medical Service
ICD	:	International Classification of Diseases
ICHPPC	:	International Classification of Health Problems in Primary Care
LHV	:	National Association of General Practitioners
LMR	:	National Medical Registration System
NIVEL	:	National Institute for Primary Health Care Research
NSAID	:	Non-Steriod Anti-Inflammatory Drug
NUHI	:	Nijmegen University General Practitioners Institute
NVRB	:	Netherlands Association for the Control of Rheumatic Diseases
POLIS	:	Outpatient Clinic Information System
RA	:	Rheumatoid Arthritis
REVIS	:	Rehabilitation Information System
SDR	:	Standard Diagnosis Registration System for Rheumatic Diseases
SIG	:	Health Care Information Centre
SIVIS	:	SIG Nursing Home Information System
STG	:	Steering Committee on Future Health Scenarios
WAGW	:	Handicapped Employees (Employment) Act
WHO	:	World Health Organization
WVC	:	Ministry of Welfare, Health and Cultural Affairs